S.95

The Story of Ruth

Also by Morton Schatzman, M.D.
SOUL MURDER: PERSECUTION IN THE FAMILY

The Story of Ruth

by Morton Schatzman, M.D.

G. P. Putnam's Sons
New York

The author gratefully acknowledges permission from the following sources to
quote material in the text:
    Hans Huber, Bern, Stuttgart, Vienna, for Hermann Rorschach,
Psychodiagnostics (plates), copyright renewed © 1948 by Hans Huber.
    Routledge & Kegan Paul Ltd. and Humanities Press, Inc., for extract from
Lectures on Psychical Research by C. D. Broad, copyright © 1962 by
C. D. Broad.

Library of Congress Cataloging in Publication Data

Schatzman, Morton.
    The story of Ruth.

    Includes bibliographical references.
    1. Rape—Psychological aspects—Case studies.
2. Child molesting—Psychological aspects—Case studies. 3. Apparitions—
Psychological aspects—Case studies. I. Title.
RC560.R36S32   616.8'521   79-20299
ISBN 0-399-12234-6

PRINTED IN THE UNITED STATES OF AMERICA

Contents

. . . Soul must become its own betrayer, its own deliverer, the one activity, the mirror turn lamp.

William Butler Yeats

Preface

I have allowed information about my personal life to be published for the sake of your understanding.

I cannot tell you where this book will lead you, but I hope it will be a key to new parts of your mind.

It was not easy for me to undergo some of the experiences described here. I had to take a trip through hell. But I survived and benefited.

I want to share with you what I have learned from my experiences.

Ruth

Introduction

THIS is a true story. Some of the incidents are extraordinary, but they actually happened. Whenever I was with Ruth, I carried a pen and paper or an audiotape machine to record what occurred. All the conversations that appear here are reported verbatim or nearly so.

Ruth came to me, a psychiatrist, because she was in a severe emotional crisis and needed help. I have pondered whether I should disclose in a book the intimacies she related to me in her therapy.

Traditionally, doctors and psychotherapists present personal facts about patients to colleagues and trainees. The education and training of professionals are considered a valid reason for disseminating confidential information. Originally, I had planned to publish various parts of this story in specialist journals, but as I proceeded with the work, I came to feel that publication should not be limited to professionals, since the issues the story deals with concern many other people. What are apparitions? Are they real? Can one trust the evidence of one's senses? And many other questions. I give case-history details with the hope that they will stimulate fresh thinking and broaden understanding about certain human experiences.

If there are people who have had experiences similar to Ruth's they are likely to find her story enlightening. They may also discover that their experiences could interest scientists, and feel encouraged to present themselves for research.

Knowing the sorts of facts the book would contain, Ruth and her husband have endorsed its publication from the time I first mentioned the idea to them.

To tell this story requires giving information about members of Ruth's family of origin. I have taken great care to disguise their real identities, and those of Ruth, her husband, and their children. If family members were to read the book, they could recognize themselves, but they would realize that no one outside the family could identify them. Nor would the family members learn much about each other that they do not already know. True, they would learn about experiences of Ruth, especially recent ones, that they had been unaware of—but she is aware of this possibility and is not worried about it.

Certain persons' behavior toward Ruth in the course of her growing up may horrify readers. Nevertheless readers might keep in mind something Ruth said to me about her past, after reading a draft of this book: "I had a very bad time of things, but I feel I've got no right to blame anyone without knowing—which I don't— all the circumstances that may have led them to act as they did."

First Meetings with Ruth

THE referral note to me from Ruth's general medical practitioner gave me no hint of the strange and remarkable events that I was soon to hear about and to witness. I reread the scrawled note just before she entered my office.

Dear Dr. Schatzman,

Twenty-five-year-old woman who requests psychiatric counselling.

Says she has been losing friends recently. "Some days I hate everybody."

Having troublesome dreams.

Provisional diagnosis: ? paranoia

? depression.

She came to my office the first time with her husband, Paul, who remained in the waiting room.

When I first saw her, nothing about her appearance or manner struck me as unusual.

I said "hello" and motioned her to a chair. "Except for your doctor's short note, I know nothing about you. Why don't you start from the beginning?"

I looked at her now more closely. She wore no makeup that I could detect. Her hair, though not untidy, had not been freshly combed for the appointment. She had on a necklace of opaque beads, a wedding ring, another ring on her right hand with a stone, and no wristwatch. A long-sleeved, light-green wool sweater matched darker green trousers. Her leather shoes were neither shiny nor scruffy. I judged her to be about twenty pounds too heavy.

She began to speak, and I started to take notes. "For four or five months now I've been feeling and acting strangely. I'm just not me. It's been hard for me to cope."

"What's been strange?"

"The first thing I noticed was feeling dirty when Paul and I tried to have sex. Paul's my husband. When he comes near to me now, I don't feel loved or good anymore, just violated and penetrated. And I can't keep those feelings from him, or just lie there pretending."

Her voice was pleasant and calm, and didn't quaver. The accent was obviously American, but I found it hard to place, since it was not typically New England, Middle Atlantic, or Southern, the accents I knew best.

"We'd had some troubles, different ones, in the first two years of marriage, but for the next six years, things had been all right, until now."

"What have you done about it?"

"I told my friend Polly about it and she said she thinks it happens to everyone who's been married for a while. She's been married twice. She gave me some pornographic magazines, dirtier than you can get in a bookstore. She said, 'Read these before you go to bed, and you'll get excited.' They did excite me a little, but they also made me feel more standoffish about sex. Since then, the problem has gotten worse. Now I can't even stand Paul's touching me."

The way she looked at me when she said these things betrayed neither pride nor shame, only a sense of pain and puzzlement.

I thought of inviting Paul to join us, but I decided not to. She might be discussing sexual matters first, not because they were the most important, but because they were the most outward expression of another, more basic, problem.

She shifted position in her chair, and went on talking. "Over the past few months I've been feeling scared. When my husband leaves the house, I'm afraid to answer the door or open it. If a neighbor, or anyone, knocks on the door I feel dread. If I go to the door, even if it's someone I know and like, I shake. I'm used to having a lot of people around, and I'm lonely if they're not. But now I don't want to see anyone. I've been locking all the doors at home, so even my children know something is wrong."

"Can you tell me your children's names and ages? That way you can refer to them and I'll know who you'll mean."

The change of subject didn't disconcert her. "George, the oldest, is seven. Heather is three. The baby, Yvonne, is fifteen months. I'm afraid to leave the house. George told his teacher that I wouldn't come out of the house because I'm sick in the head. I can't go to the bank or go shopping. I'm so afraid. When I'm out, I feel faint and fuzzy, as if my stomach is badly upset. Last time I was shopping, the store had no windows. I had to get out. I went to the car and lay my head down on the seat, until my husband, who'd also been shopping, came back. I felt ashamed and humiliated when I saw myself through his eyes. Still, he made me feel better.

"I'm afraid of doors, and crowds, and public places. The first time I noticed it I was sitting in a café drinking tea, and the conversations going on around me made me nervous. I had to get up and leave. That was embarrassing, because I got up while people were talking to me. And I didn't just walk out—I ran.

"I've never felt like this before. I don't know what's happening. I think I'm going crazy."

I responded to the last remark with only a slight raising of my eyebrows. She hadn't asked me a direct question. Besides, I didn't have enough information yet to form an adequate judgment. I asked about other fears.

Before the previous few months, she had never experienced fears of crowds, open or closed spaces, elevators, planes, or people. The only feeling even vaguely resembling any of the recent fears was an aversion to wearing a bathing cap while swimming underwater or diving. She would feel smothered. However, she had been a good swimmer, had liked swimming, and even this "fear," she said, had been more a feeling of discomfort than a fear.

From her choice of words so far, I found it hard to tell when her formal education had ended, but I guessed that she was probably not a college graduate.

She seemed to be finding relief in telling her story. For the moment, all she wanted of me was that I pay attention, and ask an occasional question.

"Apart from feeling worried about what's been happening," I asked, "have you been feeling sad?"

"Yes, very." She took a deep breath. It seemed at once to be a sigh and a reaching for more energy. "I've been getting worse lately. I've been unhappy in my life before, but I've always been able to pull myself out of it." Another deep breath. "Now I can't control my moods or what I'm feeling. I cry a lot. When I'm alone, some days I spend all day crying. I don't even clean the house anymore."

Some women, when telling me of their crying spells, start to cry. But she did not. I wondered if she had ever been punished for trying to win sympathy through tears.

"I'm feeling too many demands. I can't spread myself out far enough to do it all. I'm alone and lost. I can't bear to be in the same room as my children. I don't tend to them anymore. When my baby wakes up and cries, I feel like pushing a chest of drawers against my door. That feeling is so intense that I have to make myself not do it. It's especially there when I wake up in the morning and hear the children. I feel, Oh, my God, I don't want to open my door to them. I don't want to face another day, to start all over again. Sometimes I feel like running away. And other times I feel there is nowhere to go. I feel so guilty about my feelings toward the children, and about not cleaning the house. The more guilty I feel, the more depressed I get, the more neglectful I am."

Then, without waiting for a question, a sound, or even a gesture from me, she brought up a fresh matter.

"Have you ever had anyone tell you their brain was going to explode?"

"Yes, I have."

She ignored my answer. Perhaps she had asked because she thought she was very odd for having such an experience.

"I feel I have so much inside me that I'll keep swelling until the top blows off. I make my husband rub the top of my head to see if it's swelling. He can't convince me it's not. It feels like the bones there are coming apart."

A sensation of swelling in the head sometimes occurs in clinical depression. Yet, she didn't display certain other features of depression, such as sadness in her face or sluggishness in her speech or movements.

"Which part of the day or night is worst for you?"

"It's all bad." She sighed.

"Have you been feeling like doing harm to yourself?"

"Sometimes I really want to die. At times I feel I'm finished, and the only way out for me is to die. I want no one to have to see my body later. All I need is a good plan—which I don't have. It scares me when I think of it. But I also think that if this is what living is, I don't want to waste my time doing it. I feel guilty about dying and leaving the children, but sometimes I feel I just have to. I wish I'd never had children, so that if I died, I wouldn't have to leave them without a mother."

"How's your appetite been?"

Being questioned did not make her nervous; she seemed as comfortable now as she had earlier when telling her own story. "It's gone. I've lost twelve pounds in two weeks. When I eat, my stomach knots up. Before this, I'd vomit only if I ate something I didn't like or if I saw someone else vomit, but now I have trouble keeping any food down. I've never had vomiting spells like this before."

"Your bowels?"

"Normal." She paused, and stared at me. "I thought I had everything I wanted. I don't know why this is happening."

Again there wasn't a direct question. Perhaps "I don't know why" meant "Why?" Again I didn't answer. I had no answer.

I would shortly discover that much had been occurring which I could not have suspected.

"Have you been seeing anyone else about your troubles?"

"No—only the doctor who referred me to you, for about fifteen minutes."

"Have you tried helping yourself in some way, such as by taking pills or meditating?"

"I don't like pills, and I don't know anything about meditation."

"Have you tried using alcohol?"

"No. I wouldn't like to become dependent on it."

I was about to ask her about her sleep and the "troublesome dreams" mentioned in the doctor's note, when she said, "I've been having dreams of a sort I've never had before. I've often felt uneasy about going to sleep in complete darkness, and I usually keep a hall light on. But I've never been afraid of sleep before. Now, I'll stay up late talking, just in order not to go to sleep. I want to know why I'm dreaming the dreams and how not to be nervous about them or to care about them. Mainly, I'd like to stop dreaming them."

"Can you tell me any of your dreams?"

"I've dreamed more than once of cutting my wrist, with the blood running over my hand. In the dream I'm careful to cut my wrist lengthwise, so that it can't be fixed." She was wrong to think a lengthwise cut could not be fixed, but I did not correct her. "Then I feel better and my confusion is gone. In the dream I feel that's the answer. But when I wake up, the dream concerns me."

"Any other dreams?"

"Yes, the first one I started to have worries me even more. I'm not sure it's really a dream, because in the dream I wake up. What I mean is, I dream I wake up. There's a numb, tingling feeling that starts in my feet. It's as if my feet are going to sleep. The feeling isn't unpleasant. I wiggle my feet—or, rather, I dream I do. Then the feeling spreads up my legs, up my body, to my lips. My tongue gets thick and heavy. I panic. At this point, I realize that I'm not awake, that I'm dreaming—or I dream I realize it. I feel my tongue hanging out. I feel my tongue, and somehow at the same time I watch it. My lips feel enormous. I try to speak or scream, but only heavy sounds, in an awful voice, come out of my mouth. Then I awaken.

"This dream has been happening every night for at least a week, sometimes a few times a night. There have been nights when I'd seem to dream it every time I fell asleep. The dream doesn't start as a nightmare, but it always ends as one. It's always the same dream, but it seems to be getting stronger. It's gotten more and more gory.

"At the point in the dream when I start to talk or scream, blood from my mouth spatters all over the ceiling and walls. It feels just like vomiting or retching. It's strange because the beginning of the dream is a good sensation. And then it ends up like that.

"I've dreamed it so much now, that when it begins, I know how it's going to go on and on and end. I'll lie there, knowing I have to go through it all before I can wake up. I can't wake myself before the end.

"For the first few days I didn't tell the dream to anyone, but then I told my husband. If Paul is home during the day, I'll lie down and sleep for an hour or two. If he's working, I can't, for fear of the dream.

"At night the dream keeps waking me up. I'm not getting any sleep that amounts to anything. And I'm tired all day. That makes it even harder for me to face my children early in the morning."

We had been together now for about fifty minutes. Usually my sessions are about an hour, though I vary the time for a first consultation depending upon how much time someone seems to need. I leave myself anywhere up to two hours. I decided not to start winding up the session, since she obviously had much more to say.

As if sensing my thoughts, she announced, "I haven't told you the worst yet."

One reason for which people come to psychotherapy is to tell the therapist the worst about themselves—the worst experiences of their lives, the worst thoughts they have ever had, the worst act they have ever committed. They often narrate it on the first or second visit. They may not know before they come that this is what they want to do, and only discover it in the therapist's office. They seem to want another person to hear the worst about themselves, and to maintain nonetheless a belief in their basic worth.

"A few nights after that dream began to happen, another dream started. I had it less often but it disturbed me even more. For you to understand its meaning, I have to tell you first about something in my childhood. When I was ten my mother had a baby girl."

"How many brothers and sisters do you have altogether?"

"Mallory, a girl, is five and a half years older than me, and Andrew, a boy, is four years older, I was next, and then this girl, Jane, when I was ten.

"Jane was born in the morning, in a hospital. The next night while I was asleep in my room at home, my father entered my bedroom and woke me up. He asked me if I loved him. I said I did when he wasn't drunk, but he frightened me when he was drunk."

"Was he drunk then?"

"I'm not sure. I think not. He said everything would be different now, and he was going to be good to me. He was sitting on the side of my bed. It was a hot night, and I was only wearing panties. I remember him taking off his trousers. I couldn't see him well because it was dark. I don't recall what happened next—there's a blank—but then I remember him trying to pull down my panties and me holding on to them to stop him. Then he lay on top of me. He tried to get inside me, but I was too small. I rolled over onto my tummy to prevent him. He fought me. He rolled me onto my back and bit my nipples until they bled. He tried to put his thing into my mouth. He put it to my lips but I kept them closed. I tried to roll over again and get out of bed. I also threatened to tell my mother. He said if I did he'd kill me. He hit me on the face. I could see his fist coming, but I couldn't feel it then, though it sure hurt afterward. I remember my lip and my nose were bleeding. I could taste the blood.

"The next I recall was feeling something wet on the side of my face. It was horrible. I suppose now it was his orgasm, but I thought then he must be peeing on me.

"I didn't know at the time why he finally stopped attacking me. I just lay in bed hurting.

"I was badly bruised, and afterward it hurt when I tried to pee. Somehow I was left feeling that he hadn't hurt me enough for his own satisfaction.

"When my mother came home from the hospital I told her what had happened. I showed her the bruises. My father told her I'd been out in the playground and had been beaten up by the boys. My mother said I should never tell anyone else what I'd told her, or my father would go to jail for the rest of his life. Yet she also said she didn't believe me!"

I winced at this last disclosure.

"My mother kept on saying she didn't believe me, but decided that my father and I couldn't go on living in the same house. She told me either my father or me would have to leave. She said it was my choice, but she also said she'd vowed to God to stay with my father and didn't want to break her vow. And then I said something back to her."

"What was that?"

"I can't say."

"Why not?"

"Because I shouldn't have said it."

"But that was many years ago, and you were only a child, and in a most unpleasant and difficult situation. Nothing you might have said then would be a mark against you now—or would it?"

"All right. I said, 'Oh, why don't you and Daddy stuff it?'"

"Is that all? You'd just been attacked by your father, and your mother was asking you to leave home, almost as if it had been your fault. Under such circumstances, was what you'd said so bad?"

"I guess not, but I felt it was then."

She resumed her narrative. "I left home. I stayed at a friend's house for a few weeks. Then I was sent to a children's home where I lived for the next seven years. I'd visit my family on special occasions such as holidays, or when my father wasn't home."

"Did you ever discuss with anyone in the family what your father had done?"

"My father always denied the whole thing. He would say I'd dreamed it up. When I was grown up I asked Mallory, my older sister, if daddy ever tried to fool with her. She said no. I told her about the rape. She believed me.

"I've wondered why he'd chosen me to attack rather than Mallory. At the time of the rape she was fifteen, well-developed, and beautiful; she'd won beauty contests at school. Maybe it was because I was weaker and easier to overcome. I know now I'd done nothing to make him act that way, and there was no way I could have prevented what happened. But still it hurts. I felt singled out; I don't like that."

"He never tried anything later on with your sister who was born that day?"

"He did. Mallory told me that once, when Jane was about twelve—he was drunk—he threw her down on the sofa and asked her to give him a little. She ran away to Mallory's house. He ran after her, but he couldn't get her."

Her tale was now raising several issues in my mind that I would continue to consider after the end of the session. Could I be certain that the father's attack upon Ruth had really occurred? I wanted to know if she could tell the difference between something

actually seen, heard, or felt and something imagined or dreamed.
I felt sure that such events as she had described do happen; besides having read about them I had been told about them in my office by mothers and fathers, as well as by daughters. Ruth's father's later attempt at sexual relations with Jane was compatible with his sexual attack upon Ruth. I recalled Sigmund Freud's views about his patients' stories of having been sexually seduced and assaulted in childhood.[1] He had become convinced that his patients' stories were fantasies, and that the seductions and assaults had never actually happened; he believed his patients had invented stories of others' sexual interest in themselves to fend off memories of their own childhood erotic feelings. A problem with Freud's position, I recognized, is that although he had ascribed an interesting motive to his patients for inventing their stories, he had furnished no evidence that the stories were actually inventions. I also reasoned that even if one supposed Freud to be correct about his own patients' stories, one could not thereby assume such stories from other patients to be fantasies. There are many reported experiences that one cannot be certain correspond to actual events. People can lie and can also deceive themselves. It is helpful to have access to an independent source of evidence such as either a written record dating from near the time of the declared happening, or someone else's testimony. In Ruth's case there was nothing in writing, and the only avowed witness to the event besides her was the father, who had had no reason to corroborate her narrative and much reason to deny it. I trusted Ruth's story, since I felt no reason not to. Had she made up her tale, I thought, she would have to have also concocted the bleeding, the pain, the bruises, and her mother having seen the bruises, and her father having acknowledged them.

The mother's decision that Ruth and the father could not go on living in the same house implied that the mother believed Ruth's story. Why, then, had she professed disbelief? Perhaps she had been so dependent upon her husband emotionally or financially that she had felt she could not afford to admit believing Ruth. Perhaps she had feared a scandal. Perhaps she had feared he would be violent. Perhaps she had had sexual experiences that she had felt guilty about and thought she was not in a position to criticize. Perhaps, as she had told Ruth, she had really vowed to God to stay with her husband and wished to keep her vow. Whatever her reasons, I knew it was not uncommon, when a woman is aware that her husband and daughter have had sexual relations, for the woman to keep quiet about them—even if those sexual relations are ongoing.

I also knew it is not unusual for a child who is the victim of an adult's sexual attack to feel guilty, as if it were somehow the child's fault. Ruth might have been especially likely to feel this way, given her mother's interest in protecting the father. Apparently Ruth had received no sympathy or support from anyone.

I wondered about the sort of person the father was and about his motives. Was his behavior expressing a general sexual preference for prepubertal girls (that is, might he be regarded as a sexual deviant or pervert), or was it expressing a form of behavior that was acceptable within his social group? The mother's response made me question whether she rejected his behavior altogether, even if she saw it as a problem. Had he been sexually frustrated? Had his wife withdrawn from him, and thereby deserted him in a sense? Perhaps he had experienced her being away to deliver a baby as a desertion.

Why had he been violent? Had he tried first to induce Ruth to submit to him sexually by promises or by prevailing upon her wish to please him, and failed? Or had he used violence because he preferred to subjugate her brutally rather than bribe her or persuade her by other means?

Why had he chosen Ruth rather than Mallory? It occurred to me that Ruth had been too young to have become pregnant, whereas Mallory had not. Was this his reason? Or was Ruth right in thinking he had selected her because she had been easier to overpower?

His behavior suggested that he was unaware of how humiliated and bewildered he made her feel, or, if he was aware, that he was willing—or even perhaps wanting—to make her feel that way.

Ruth and I could not have anticipated at this time that we were to acquire more information about the incident and also were to gain a fresh perspective about it. These we would attain by a most unusual means, which we had no inkling would become available to us. But I am getting ahead of the story. Suffice to say at this point that her dreams were not the means we used.

She continued her narrative. "From then on, during my teenage years and after I got married, my father and I had a distant, polite relationship. Just after I gave birth to Heather—I was twenty-two—my mother phoned to say my father was coming to visit us as a houseguest. Paul and I were still living in America."

"How long have you been in England?"

"About two years. Paul's company transferred him here. My father was going to build a crib for the baby and do any other carpentry around the house we might need, and was also going to give us some money. I was worried, because for part of that time Paul was going to be away on a business trip. I discussed the situation with Paul. Paul was a little concerned. He said if there was any trouble, I should phone him, and he'd come home right away.

"When my father came I was cautious. I didn't like his being around. He slept in George's room, while my son slept with me. The first day or two passed all right. Then, one night I awoke and saw my father standing in the room. He'd been drinking. He hugged me and asked me why I didn't show him affection. He went down on his knees and asked me if I recalled that night when I was ten. He told me he loved me. He said he'd always loved me, he'd always been sexually attracted to me, he hadn't been able to stand not being able to touch me as a little girl, he hadn't been happy with my mother because of it, he'd like to go away with me, and—if I wouldn't—he'd like to hug and kiss me and have me respond to him once.

"I picked up my children, one in each arm, and drove to a phone booth. I phoned Paul. He said he'd come home. He advised me to sleep at the home of some friends of ours. I phoned my mother too. She said, 'Don't phone the police.' Then I phoned the friends, who put me and the children up for the night. When Paul got home he was annoyed with himself for not having stopped my father from coming in the first place. He changed the locks on the door, because I'd given my father a house key. After that, my father disappeared and didn't return to my mother for six months.

"About two years ago, I was visiting my family. I was going to take my sister Jane swimming. I arrived at my parents' home wearing a swimsuit covered on top with a shirt. My father appeared in the kitchen, while no one else was in the room, and put his hand down the back of my swimsuit. Somehow that seemed typical of him. If I went back there now, he might try it again.

"When I tell you these things, I feel filthy and dirty. I feel ugly to be remembering all this. I feel ashamed for my father."

I replied, "Yet you are telling me, which may indicate that you want someone else, perhaps especially someone outside the family, to know. What about the dream you'd wanted to tell me that you said has been bothering you?"

"In that dream I'm a little girl. The room is dark." Ruth's eyes became tearful. "I sense someone's presence. I don't know what happens next, but then my father is in bed with me, hurting me. He has a terrible smile on his face. I feel his hands on my thighs and knees, pulling them apart. In my dream, he has complete sexual intercourse with me, which he didn't in real life. It's painful. Blood splashes up out of my vagina.

"I awaken terrified. I look at my husband and see my father where my husband is lying. I know the man in bed is Paul even while I'm seeing my father but the man I see is my father. I can see my father's face whenever I think about the dream and even when I don't think about it. Sometimes, in the daytime, I look at Paul and for a moment he seems to look like my father."

I was aware that a dream can bring the dreamer back to a disturbing experience that occurred years earlier in waking life, and that such a dream sometimes repeats itself. I know too that, for some moments after waking, one may occasionally continue to see a figure that has been present in a dream. Sometimes the distressing scenes and emotions of a nightmare may persist for hours or days.

She went on: "Once, recently, I dreamed of Paul raping me. In the dream, I hurt and bled. Then I was somehow running, and was afraid. There were things spinning around, like the spokes of a wheel. I awoke and couldn't figure out where I was or who anyone was. I can't make any sense of the dream—Paul is gentle, and has never been physically violent with me during lovemaking or otherwise."

I said, "Maybe what you've just been telling me is connected with the sexual difficulties you described at the start."

She said nothing. Then she asked, "Do you think I'm crazy?"

"No. I think you're undergoing a severe emotional crisis but you seem sane to me."

"That's a relief."

"I'd like to discuss the situation with your husband and you together."

I went to fetch Paul from the waiting room.

He was reading a psychology textbook he had brought with him. I wondered if his interest in it was related to Ruth's condition or to something else.

Having followed the direction of my gaze, he grinned. "I'm taking a management course," he said. "That's why I'm reading this."

He stood up and shook my hand. He was about the same age as his wife, perhaps two or three years older, and was dressed tastefully in a sport jacket, colored shirt, and tie.

I motioned him toward the office.

When we entered, she said to me, "Do I need to go into a hospital?"

"I think you could use a rest, a vacation from housework and from your children. I'm recommending that you go to the Arbours Crisis Centre for a week or two."

Arbours is an organization in London which I, Dr. Joseph Berke, and other friends set up in 1971.[2] It is registered in the United Kingdom as a charity and exists to provide help and places to live outside mental hospitals for people in emotional distress. In 1974 Arbours created a Crisis Centre where individuals, couples, or families who are in crisis can live for limited periods of time and receive intensive care and attention. The Centre is an ordinary house in a quiet residential neighborhood. We call the people who stay there guests, not patients. They come to the Centre only if they choose to; they come and go as they please while staying there; they receive no therapy—such as drugs—against their wills; and they participate themselves in the decision about when they will leave the Centre.

I explained about the Crisis Centre to Ruth and Paul. "I think the Centre might be right for you," I told her. "You could get a good rest there if someone suitable were found to look after the children. And while you're there, you could see me every day."

"I do want to get away from it all," she said. "With everything I've been going through, it's been more than I can tolerate. What do you think, Paul?"

"I'd agree to do anything that could help."

"Do either of you have any idea what might have brought Ruth's condition about?" I asked.

Ruth and Paul looked at each other and back at me without changing their facial expressions.

"What sort of thing could have?" Paul asked.

"A physical illness, surgery, the loss of someone important to Ruth, a drop in income, moving house, some new worry or responsibility, or some other upsetting life event. Maybe even a success that Ruth might be finding it hard to adjust to."

Again they looked at each other, for a longer time than before, and back at me.

"No, none of those things," Ruth said.

"So that means that your condition isn't a reaction to an external stress," I said. I made a noise with closed lips indicating a mixture of puzzlement and satisfaction with that conclusion.

I asked some questions to find out if Ruth had suffered from a mental disorder before the previous few months, and Paul's and Ruth's answers indicated that she had not.

"As you've been feeling both depressed and nervous lately," I said to Ruth, "you might consider taking an antidepressant drug and perhaps a sedative." I explained to her what drugs were available, what each drug's principal effects were known to be, and which of her recent experiences each might be likely to help her cope with.

"I don't like the idea of taking pills, but I will if you think it'll help."

We decided that Ruth would come to the Centre in eight days, which would give her and Paul time to make arrangements for the children, and that in those eight days I would see her twice more.

Paul and Ruth left my office.

"I've told you that when I look at Paul I sometimes see my father's face," she began at our second session, "but that's not all. Sometimes even when I've been awake, I've seen my father as I've been looking at Yvonne who's fifteen months. Yvonne cries and wakes me up. It may be that I've been having a nightmare. I go to her to pick her up and hold her. I reach down to her crib to get her, and see my father's face. His face is upon hers. I hear him laughing and her crying, but his laugh is smothering her crying sounds. I want to reach out to her. But I'd be touching *him*, so I'm afraid to reach for her.

"One night recently I had a dream just like this. In the dream it's nighttime. I can hear Yvonne crying as if she needs me. I get up and go to her room. I turn on the light and look into her crib. I see Yvonne's body, but my father's head. My father has a horrible smile and is laughing at me. He's laughing, because he knows he's gotten into my dream. Yvonne is crying, but her crying is somehow underneath him, as if he's put his face on top of hers. I can hear her but I can't touch her."

She also said, "I've taken one of the sedative pills, but I don't see how they can help me. I'm not going to take any more."

I chose not to press the matter.

"I haven't told you everything," she said at the next session. "When I'm alone in the house, I feel there is someone else in the room with me, who wants me to die. I feel I'm in terrible danger and should leave my house—right away! I wish I could run. But I can't go, because my children are with me. It feels like something terrible is there with me."

"You say you feel someone else is in the room with you, and you also speak of some*thing* terrible. Is there a person or a thing?"

"It's foolish to say it's my father's presence. I know my father is alive and is thousands of miles away. He isn't in my house with me. Yet I feel as if he is. I feel he wants me to die. Maybe I should die."

She told me that whenever she entered my office she was thinking, Well, this is it. This time he'll probably decide I'm crazy and he'll have me in a straitjacket inside an ambulance on the way to a mental hospital.

"That's not what I've been thinking," I replied. "You've been having some unusual and frightening experiences, but you've responded sanely to them. Any reasonable person would worry if she were having the experiences you've been having."

Later she said, "Sometimes my father's face and voice are there when I look at someone else but at other times he appears on his own. Even now, when I look at you, I can see that face from my dreams, my father's face. If you weren't who you are—if you were a friend or a neighbor—I'd tell you to leave, or I'd leave myself."

I was beginning to understand that her dreams, her seeing her father when awake, and the symptoms of distress that she had previously narrated to me were all connected.

I wondered whether her fear of being thought crazy had kept

her from disclosing to me other strange experiences she might have been having.

The fourth session was our first at the Arbours Crisis Centre. There Ruth told me of a most unusual experience she had had at home one morning, a few days before she had first come to see me.

"I had been awake for some minutes. I was turning the corner of the living room on my way through the dining room into the kitchen. There my father was, sitting at the dining-room table. He was drinking a cup of coffee and laughing. At first I thought he'd arrived from America, and I'd been having those bad dreams in anticipation of his coming. This thought lasted a moment. Then I realized it couldn't be him because he didn't have enough money to make the trip, and also, because the doors to the house were locked. At some point I may have asked, 'What are you doing here?' but I can't honestly say. He looked so real that if this had happened in my hometown, I'd have probably sat down and had a cup of coffee with him.

"I ran to the bedroom, woke Paul, and said, 'Paul, I've seen my daddy sitting at the dining-room table.' He just said, 'Oh.' I said, 'Go look.' And then I changed my mind, and said I'd look again myself. If my father was still there, and if Paul would look and not see him, I'd want Paul to get me to a doctor quickly. A lot of worrying things had been happening to me and I'd avoided going to a doctor. And seeing someone who wasn't there would be the last straw.

"I looked, and he was there. Paul looked, and didn't see anybody. I started to cry, and I said, 'Paul, I know this is crazy.' He put his arm around me and said, 'Maybe you're just a little bit crazy.' He said people who were just a little bit crazy could get better. Then he went and looked a second time and saw no one. I said, 'I don't think I've ever been crazy before, Paul.' He said, 'Well, maybe you're just a little bit, but I love you anyway.'

"I was still seeing my father in the dining room. I would look in there, and—this is just like the old buzzard—he'd grin and wave

his hand at me. He'd have a knowing expression on his face—
'knowing' in the sense of knowing I was the only one who could
see him. I'd say, 'Paul, it's still there.'

"My father appeared to me many times after that. I'd see him in
various rooms, at all times of day or night. It was like he was living
with us. I knew he couldn't possibly really be there, but I'd see
him, hear him walking around, and see and hear him opening and
closing doors. This experience frightened me more than anything
else. I'd get especially upset when I'd see him walking into
Yvonne's room. All the time I'd be telling myself, 'This is crazy.
There isn't anyone there. There couldn't be.' Do you still think
I'm not crazy?"

"I don't think you're crazy, though it's a very strange experience."

"When he appears, I feel he's wanting me to do away with
myself. Sometimes I feel he's telling me I'm going to die. He might
do something to me—like pushing me in front of a train or pulling
out a knife and stabbing me. I also worry about what I might do to
myself, just to get away from him. He doesn't tell me to slash my
wrists, but when I see him or am about to see him, I feel like
doing it. If I killed myself, he'd leave. That's the only way he'll
leave me alone, I think. And he's not going to give up until he's
seen me do it."

The next day, she unfolded more of the story. "Just before I
came to the Crisis Centre, I was feeling better, more optimistic,
because I'd met you. I was hoping you'd help me work things out.
Two ladies who were going by my house knocked on my door to
say hello. I invited them in for coffee, as a kind of self-therapy.

"They went to the dining room and sat down. I had already
made some coffee. In the kitchen I poured it from the pot into a
serving jug. Then I put the jug, three cups, three spoons, a small
pitcher of milk, a little bowl of sugar, a few napkins, and a plate of
cookies onto a tray, and carried the tray into the dining room.

"There was a chair between the two ladies, and my father was
sitting in it. I saw him, and my hands started to tremble. A bit of

coffee and some milk spilled on the tray. One of the ladies, Suzanne, asked, 'Ruth, what on earth is wrong with you?' I didn't want them to know. I said, 'I haven't been feeling well.' My hands were trembling so much that Suzanne stood up to help me. My father turned to her and said, 'Don't worry, I'll get the tray.' I just stood there with my mouth open, fascinated and frightened. Suzanne didn't hear him, and she took the tray.

"I sat there trying to have coffee. The other lady asked me if I was pregnant. I said, 'No, every time someone gets sick it doesn't mean they're pregnant.' She said, 'I've noticed your house isn't getting cleaned lately.'

"Meanwhile, I was looking at my father. The two ladies didn't know he was there, but he was following the talk, looking and nodding at whoever was speaking. Every so often he would look at me and grin, and wave his hand at me. He knew he was upsetting me; he meant to upset me.

"After a little while I told the ladies I wasn't feeling well and they'd have to leave. I was afraid of being left alone with my father, but I didn't let it show. I just let them leave."

She paused and looked at me, waiting, I supposed, to see how I'd respond. I was fascinated, but I said nothing.

She continued. "I hope I won't see him here at the Crisis Centre. It's been twenty-four hours and I haven't seen him, either when I've been awake or in my dreams."

As it turned out, her hope was soon frustrated.

In her sixth session—her third since coming to the Centre—she said, "I wonder if my father allowed me that day of freedom just to show me he could be good if he wanted to."

"Oh?"

"Last evening, when we were all sitting around in the kitchen, he appeared. He was outside in the back garden near the kitchen door. I could see him through the glass panel of the door. He just stood there watching and laughing. It was raining, and he was standing in the rain, but it didn't seem to bother him, which struck me as funny. His presence frightened me. He didn't act as if he were going to come in, yet I was afraid he would, and I'd have to talk to him in front of other people. I left the kitchen without telling anyone why I was leaving. I didn't want anyone in the house to know I was seeing a person who wasn't there.

"When I went up to my room I tried to forget about him, but I couldn't. I went to sleep and started to dream of him. He was standing at the foot of my bed smiling. I woke up frightened and felt terribly sad. I cried until I fell asleep again.

"Then I dreamed of being a little girl staying here at the Crisis Centre, and of being happy. An aunt of mine comes in late at night and says she has come to fetch me. In the next scene I'm still a little girl. I'm back with my parents, and my father is drunk. He's coming toward me saying he's going to kill the 'goddamned little bastard'—meaning me. I try to get back to the Crisis Centre. Then I woke up. I assured myself it was a dream, and went back to sleep. I dreamed again I was at home, trying to get back to the Centre. Again I woke up. Finally I stopped dreaming.

"This morning I awoke from another dream and saw my father standing there laughing. I could feel the bed moving from his legs knocking against it. I felt as if he was threatening to kill me, just as he had in my dream. I awoke trembling, my legs were shaking, and my stomach was knotted. It was worse than having the flu.

"If I see my father everywhere I must be a nut.

"I thought of packing my bags and leaving. I even looked for road maps. I'm just so frightened."

At that moment, as she was looking at a point just to the left of where I was sitting, she began to tremble and to wring her hands. The pupils of her eyes seemed to grow larger.

"He's here," she whispered.

I turned to my left to look but saw no one.

"Where?"

She pointed to the spot at which I had just looked, about eight feet from her. "He's standing there." She was trembling more than before, biting her knuckles and gasping.

Again I looked and saw no one.

"He looks as real as you do, real and fleshy. He has an ugly smile. I can see each tooth very clearly. I wish it were just a shadow, not flesh." She was pale, and very frightened. "I can hear him laughing."

"Is he saying anything?" I asked.

"No. He usually doesn't. He's just laughing, as if everything is hysterically funny."

"Since you say he's as real as I am, would it be possible for you to touch him?"

"No. It would feel too terrible."

Ruth at the Crisis Centre

RUTH's case was unique in my experience as a psychiatrist. Never before had I met or even heard of anyone whose central problem was persecution by an apparition. Neither had the colleagues whom I told about Ruth. Nevertheless I was hopeful about being able to help her. One reason was that she felt her present state of mind was very inconsistent with her usual state, up to a few months before. She was strongly motivated to rid herself of her present problems and to return, or progress, to normality.

The resident staff at the Arbours Crisis Centre consisted of Drs. Andrea Sabbadini and Laura Forti, husband and wife. Both were psychologists in their mid-twenties who had come from Italy to work at Arbours. During Ruth's stay they played a central role in helping her. They and I often discussed her case together.

I knew we could not keep Ruth long at the Centre. She and Paul knew no one who could look after their three children for long periods. Paul had taken two weeks' leave from work, which was all he could manage. He planned to spend some days with her at the Centre and some days looking after the children and the household.

From the start I had to deal with Ruth's worry that she might be "going crazy." "Isn't someone who sees things that aren't there crazy?" she had asked.

"What do you mean by 'sees things that aren't there'?" I had replied. I had thought I knew what she meant, but I wanted her to say it—which she did:

"Seeing things that no one else is seeing."

I wondered if the invisibility to other people of what she had been seeing necessarily meant that nothing was there. Was it possible she was seeing something which everyone else was blind to? I found it very difficult to conceive of the sort of object, being, or entity that no one else but her could see.

I kept these reflections to myself, not wanting to confuse her more. Instead I asked, "What do you mean by 'crazy'?"

"Out of my mind, mad, nuts—you know, crazy."

I considered her notion that she was going crazy understandable. Some psychiatrists might have agreed with her, though I did not. In a recent well-publicized study,[3] eight sane individuals—three psychologists, a psychology graduate student, a psychiatrist, a pediatrician, a painter, and a housewife—sought admission as mental patients to twelve different American hospitals. At the hospital admission offices they complained of only one symptom, which they had invented for the purposes of the study: hearing voices. They said the voices were unclear, but as far as they could tell, the voices were saying "empty," "hollow," "thud." Besides saying they heard voices, and besides falsifying their names and (in some cases) their vocations and employments, they told the truth in all details about themselves, their life histories, and their circumstances.

All eight pseudopatients were admitted to psychiatric wards. From the time they were admitted, all behaved normally and stopped asserting they were hearing voices. Yet all eight were kept in the hospital for periods from seven to fifty-two days, the average stay being nineteen days.

The psychiatrists of these eight pseudopatients kept them in the hospital for one reason alone: the pseudopatients were hallucinating. In Ruth's idiom, they were hearing things that weren't there. Seven of the eight pseudopatients were labeled "schizophrenic" on admission. This means that some psychiatrists consider the report of hallucinations alone, in the absence of any other evidence of insanity, as warranting the diagnosis "schizophrenia" and requiring admission to a mental ward.

It was therefore reasonable for Ruth to fear that I might regard her as crazy, and I had to reassure her many times that I did not. The closest translation of "crazy" in psychiatric language is "psychotic." Besides the psychoses that reflect known disorders of the body or the brain, from which she was not suffering, there are two major groups of psychoses: the schizophrenias and the depressions. Was she undergoing one of these? The American psychiatrists in the study just cited had been mistaken in labeling their pseudopatients schizophrenic. The pseudopatients had been displaying none of schizophrenia's standard manifestations. The same was true of Ruth. Hallucinations are not a primary or defining feature of schizophrenia. One can be considered schizophrenic without hallucinating and, more importantly, one can hallucinate without being regarded as schizophrenic.

Certainly Ruth was depressed, both in the lay sense of the term—feeling unhappy much of the time—and in the psychiatric sense, as she was suffering from diminished appetite, weight loss, disturbed sleep, feelings of swelling in the head, crying spells, feelings of shame and guilt, and suicidal thoughts. However, she was not depressed to a degree that would ordinarily be regarded as psychotic. For example, unlike people with a depressive psychosis, she was clear and logical in her thinking, and lively in her speech, facial expressions, and movements. She did not feel that the world was barren or that her future was hopeless.

I explained my thinking to Ruth. She supposed that the very

fact of "seeing things that aren't there" might mean that she was crazy, whether or not she fitted into a known category of craziness. I believed her to be wrong, and told her why. Firstly, she had come to a rational understanding of her strange experiences: although she perceived someone as being there, she had concluded that no real person was there. Secondly, research into the incidence of hallucinatory experiences has disclosed that it is statistically common for mentally healthy people living in Western society to have had such an experience.[4]

One group of normal people who tend to hallucinate are the bereaved. Their hallucinations recur, as Ruth's did, and are generally of one particular figure, the dead husband or wife. A widow or widower may sense the former partner's presence, speak to the partner, hear the partner's voice or footsteps, or see an apparition of the partner. These phenomena, which may persist for years, are not rare, though many people are unaware of how common they are.[5] Persons who have such experiences may at first believe they are going mad. They can often find comfort in knowing that other sane bereaved people have had similar experiences.

Ruth told me of a bereaved person in her own family who had undergone such an experience. "About nine years ago, my mother's older sister, Grace, lost her husband after a long illness. Grace was in her mid-forties. Soon after his death, Grace began to feel his presence when she lay down in bed. Then she started to see him upon waking up. She was afraid, and moved to another room to sleep. Then she began to talk to him, and felt less frightened, so she returned to sleeping in the first room. She found that it was reassuring to see him and talk to him, since it meant to her she would never be separated from him."

"So Grace changed her attitude toward an apparition," I said, "and stopped feeling frightened of it. Maybe you could too. I'd like you to consider something else. You believe that your experience of your father is probably a product of your imagination, don't you?"

"Yes."

"Has it occurred to you that you might be allowing the apparition to manifest?"

"But I don't want it to. You don't think I do want it to, do you?" she said indignantly.

"Maybe 'allowing' isn't quite the right word. I believe you could learn to have some control over its manifesting."

"I don't understand. How could I?"

"I'll explain, using a comparison. Just as you haven't thought you could influence the apparition, most people don't think it's possible to direct their own dreams. But it is possible."

I told Ruth about a tribe in Malaya called the Senoi, whose members learn from childhood to master their dream enemies.[6] The Senoi, who number twelve thousand, are primitive by our technological standards and illiterate. They spend minimal time at planting, food gathering, and other work to provide for their material needs. Their main interest is dreams. Each morning at breakfast every family member tells a dream. Children start reporting dreams as soon as they can talk, and receive praise for doing so. Adults ask the child how he or she behaved in the dream. They congratulate the child for dream behavior they believe to be correct, point out wrong dream behavior, and suggest changes for future dream behavior. After breakfast many adults go to the village council where dream symbols and situations are discussed. I described the Senoi to Ruth so that she would understand their general principle that the dreamer must confront and conquer danger in dreams. For instance, a Senoi child who reports dreaming of being pursued by a tiger might be told that a dream tiger, unlike a real one, will only chase someone who shows fear toward it. The next time that dream occurs—and the child is informed it will occur again soon—the child must turn around, face the tiger, and attack it. If the dreamer cannot prevail over the tiger, he or she should call on dream friends for help, and fight until they arrive. The dreamer is told that once the dream enemy has been confronted and conquered, it must be forced to give the dreamer a gift. The gift might be an invention, a poem, a song, a dance, a design, a story, or a solution to a problem. It must be something that the dreamer can, when awake, display to other people as having value. By the age of adolescence, a Senoi child no longer has nightmares.

I have found this Senoi principle effective with dreams of mine, of persons I have seen in therapy, and of children. When my older son Daniel was five, I told Ruth, he dreamed that two foxes attacked him and his younger brother in our living room. Daniel felt frightened. In his dream he and his younger brother jumped into their mother's arms. The foxes continued to attack. Daniel awoke in the middle of the night and told me the dream. I responded as a Senoi father would.

One morning a week later, Daniel said he had dreamed of seeing the foxes in our living room again. This time I had been there as a lion and had frightened the foxes away.

Ruth laughed when I told her this.

I praised Daniel for having transformed his dream, and suggested he dream it once again, and this time triumph over the foxes without my help. A few days later he dreamed the same scenario again, but this time he opened the door to our house, and the foxes ran out. A bus then came up the road. The door of the bus opened. The foxes ran into the bus, and he closed the door of the bus. The bus drove off.[7]

Ruth laughed again when I told her this.

I suggested he have yet another dream in which he would demand a gift from the foxes. But he refused, saying there was no point in it, as the only gifts he would want—certain toys—wouldn't exist outside the dream.

I did not know whether Ruth's father's apparition would be susceptible to her deliberate control. That the course of dreams may be influenced by their creator does not mean that the behavior of apparitions may. However, I decided to assume that she could master the apparition—without telling her that I was only assuming it—and to see what would happen. I wanted her to face and master whatever the apparition represented. I did not fully understand what the apparition meant. Why not have her face and master the apparition itself?

"Now," I said, "if one can confront and conquer a dream antagonist, the same should apply to an apparitional one. In both cases, the mind that has apparently created the antagonist should be able to take away its power or banish it."

As I was expressing these last thoughts, Ruth began to bite her fingers and to shake. She looked away from me. "I think I'd feel strange relating to a person or a thing that's unreal as if it were real," she said hesitantly.

"But you are relating to an apparition as if it were real when you fear it could push you onto train tracks."

She nodded silently in acknowledgment. She still seemed frightened. "I don't want to face that image of my father again. I just hope he never appears."

When her father appeared to her in my office, she was terrified. I have never seen anyone so overcome by fear.

"What you're seeing isn't a real person," I said, while she sat staring at the apparition. "You're real, he isn't. You can prevail over him. You should bend him to your will. He's your creation and exists only by virtue of your power to make him exist. Just as you've made him appear, you can make him disappear. He's no threat to you. No one is there for you to fear. You should concentrate on being unafraid." I talked continuously for about three minutes, repeating the same ideas and the same words in different combinations.

As I spoke, she became visibly less fearful.

"Make him tell you why he's here," I said.

"I can't," she replied weakly. She glanced at me briefly, and then looked back at the place to my left where she was seeing the apparition.

"You can and you should," I said firmly, in the tone of voice I wanted her to use in speaking to the apparition.

She continued staring at it for about half a minute.

"Why are you here?" she finally said softly, her voice quavering. "Don't beg or plead. Demand!"

She was silent. I thought she might be gathering up courage.

"What are you doing here, huh?" She said it a little more strongly, still looking at that space to my left.

She turned to me. "He's only laughing. He's not answering."

I heard no sound of laughter.

Her eyes moved slowly across the room. "He's walking toward the door. He's looking at me and still laughing . . . He's reached the door . . . and he's passing right through it. He's disappeared."

She looked relieved, but still trembled. "He gave off an odor just like my father's. I can smell it now, even though he's gone."

I could smell nothing unusual.

Her remark brought to my mind a blind man I had once heard of, who used to hallucinate the arrival of people he knew by their sounds and odors. After hallucinating the sounds of their departures, he sometimes continued to smell their odors in the room.

Ruth turned to me. "That's the first time I've ever spoken to him. Before you told me to, I'd never have dared."

"Why do you use the word 'apparition'?" Ruth asked me once. "I've been using the word 'image.'"

I had been considering the same question. "'Image,'" I said, "calls to mind an experience in imagination. When someone imagines something, one doesn't mistake it for something really there."

She nodded.

"I've thought of other words," I said. "'Ghost' suggests the spirit or soul of a dead person. But your real father is alive. 'Specter' and 'vision' both refer to something seen. Besides seeing your father, you've sensed his presence in the room, you've smelled him, and once you heard him say something to your lady guests. So 'specter' and 'vision' wouldn't cover the range of your experiences."

As Ruth seemed to follow my line of reasoning, I continued.

"'Spirit' indicates a being's animating principle, a soul, in contrast to its material elements. I haven't used this word with you, as I'm uncertain whether I believe that spirits or souls exist."

She seemed disappointed at this remark.

"'Phantasm' and 'phantom' have occurred to me too," I said. "But they imply illusion, deception, fantasy."

"You think those words don't fit my experiences?" There was a note of surprise in her voice.

"They almost certainly do." I said "almost certainly" because at moments I had wondered if what she had been experiencing might correspond with something that really was there. I knew this idea was very farfetched, and I had entertained it privately and only fleetingly. I quickly went on. "'Apparition' simply means that which appears. I think it's the best word."

I wanted Ruth to stop avoiding situations she feared, such as being on her own in public places and traveling on public transportation.[8]

"Why don't you expose yourself to situations you're frightened of?" I had said once. "When nothing bad happens, you'll prove to yourself—and to the apparition—that there's nothing to fear.

"The Crisis Centre is about forty-five minutes from my office by public transportation, and you have to change trains and walk a few minutes at each end. In going to and from our sessions, you'll have a chance to face situations you've been afraid of."

"All right," she said. "I'm scared, but I'll try."

Her agreeing to try meant to me that she was ready, or very nearly ready, for traveling on her own. Had she refused, I would not have pressed her, but would have proposed an easier task, such as taking part of the trip alone and the rest of it accompanied by someone.

Before making the trip the first time, she had been nervous. However, when she tried it and experienced no mishap, she felt reassured. The next two return journeys had been uneventful too, and she had felt more confident. She had even started walking by herself to a park that was two streets away from the Centre. On her way back to the Centre from my office the fourth time, something unusual occurred, which she and Andrea Sabbadini told me about the next day.

That fourth time—it was about twelve noon—she saw a man sitting in front of her on the train change into her father. She became frightened. When she reached her stop and got off the train, the man got off too, behind her. He had her father's form. She hoped he would walk in a different direction, but he did not. She ran to a phone at the station to call the Crisis Centre to ask someone to meet her. Andrea answered the phone.

"I'm very embarrassed to be phoning," Ruth said, "but I think a man is following me. I'm too frightened to walk the half-mile to the Centre alone. Could someone fetch me?"

"I'll come right away," Andrea replied.

While speaking on the phone, her back to the open entrance of the phone box, Ruth felt a touch on her back. It terrified her, because she thought it was the man. She was too scared to turn around to look.

Andrea went quickly to meet her. Meanwhile Ruth started walking toward the Centre. As she walked along, she heard footsteps and the rustling of trousers behind her. When she ran, the footsteps ran, and when she walked, they walked. After having walked about half the distance, she saw Andrea coming toward her. She started running toward him.

When he got close to her, he saw she was terrified, as afraid as he had ever seen anyone. He hugged her.

"A man is following me," she said.

Andrea looked and saw no one there. The street was deserted. "Where is he?" Andrea asked.

"Behind me."

"Why don't you look back and see?"

"No, I wouldn't dare. I just want to walk straight home."

After they had walked awhile, Andrea asked if her follower was still there.

"Yes, I can hear him."

"Look back."

"No."

"It's important that you look."

She turned her head a little. "He's gone away," she said.

Because she hesitated as she said it, and did not turn her head all the way around, Andrea disbelieved her. "You said he's gone just so that I'll stop asking you to look back."

Five minutes later she admitted the footsteps were still there. When she and Andrea arrived home, her follower was gone.

Later she said to me, "About the touch I felt on my back when making that phone call: I wonder if I hallucinated it or if that man had noticed how upset I was and had approached me and actually touched me to reassure me. What do you think?"

"I don't know. I do know you survived that experience, however frightened you were. You've shown that you can bear the fear and that if you do so, the apparition will eventually disappear. I'd like you to keep making the trip back and forth to my office."

"All right."

That had not been her last fright of the day.

"A few hours later," she told me, "as I was leaving my bedroom, I saw my father in the hall. I returned to my bedroom. I felt I couldn't face him. I'd had enough for one day—or so I thought.

"In the evening, I was in the living room reading a book. There he was again, lying on the sofa. He was smiling cheerfully, not laughing as he sometimes does. His smiling seemed to say that I could do nothing about his being there, just as I hadn't been able to in my own home. I wouldn't let him matter, I said to myself, as he wasn't really there."

I nodded approvingly.

"I kept on reading. I told myself I wasn't frightened, but he said I was. I heard his voice, as if someone in the room was talking."

"It's unusual for you to hear him, isn't it?"

"I've heard him laugh and I've heard footsteps, but usually he doesn't speak."

"What happened next?"

"I tried to read, but couldn't. Then I heard him open the living-room door, walk out, and close the door behind him. I didn't look up. I listened to hear him leave the house, but I heard nothing.

"I don't like him to see me as weak." She trembled a bit as she said that. "I feel such rage toward him. He's responsible for my being weak in the first place. I'm also afraid of his gaining confidence from my weakness. I'm in a battle with him. I've put up a strong fight, and got ahead. But now I feel he's got the upper hand and will win in the end."

"What's the fight about? What will he win?"

"Me. I'm what the fight is about. It's about mastery or possession of me. I'm afraid of his getting control of me or even becoming me."

The next day, she told me another tale. Andrea also gave me his version.

After returning to the Centre from her session with me, she had gone out for a walk. As it was raining, she went upstairs when she got back to comb her hair. When she had entered her bedroom, her father was sitting on her bed. She turned around and went downstairs, where Laura was, and remained there a few hours.

Later, before going upstairs again, she told Laura, "My father was upstairs earlier, and I felt frightened."

"I'll go upstairs with you," Laura replied.

"Don't bother. That was a few hours ago."

She went upstairs to her bedroom. Her father was sitting on her bed, in a different position than before. He smelled as though he had not bathed for a few days. The odor was so strong she could smell it from the doorway. "In other words," she told me, "he stank!"

She turned away and knocked on the door of Laura and Andrea's room. Andrea was sitting at his desk.

Ruth said to him, "I'm sorry to disturb you . . ."

Andrea saw she was in the same state as when he'd met her coming from the train station.

". . . But my father is sitting on my bed."

"All right, we'll go and see," Andrea suggested.

"Why don't *you* go and see?"

"Let's go together."

Reluctantly, she went with him. When he opened the door to her room, she jumped back.

"Is he still there?" Andrea asked.

"Yes." She pointed to her pillow.

To show that her father was not there, Andrea sat on the pillow. If he could sit on the pillow, he reasoned, her father could not really be there.

However, she looked away. "I can't bear to look," she said.

Andrea moved to another part of the bed.

Again she saw her father on the pillow, and was terrified.

"Sit down next to me," Andrea said.

She did, trembling with fear.

He took her hand and held it. "Let's have a talk with your father," he said. "All right?"

"All right."

"Ask him what he wants from you."

She stared silently for about half a minute toward the head of the bed. "He says I know what he wants," she said.

"How did he know what your question was without your speaking aloud?"

She turned to Andrea. "I've found he reads my thoughts."

"Ask him why he's persecuting you."

She stared again at the apparition. "He says that I'm a bastard, that he wants me to die, and that he'll persecute me until I do die."

"Ask him why he wants you to die."

Once more she stared. "He says I know why . . . he refuses to say more." She was getting increasingly agitated and frightened.

Andrea felt he had to try again to persuade her that the apparition was unreal and that she could choose to rid herself of it. Still holding her hand, he went on. "You must understand that there really isn't anyone here besides you and me. Your father isn't really here. Because he's not really here, he can't harm you, so you needn't be afraid."

"It's hard for me to hear what you're saying. My father's speaking again, and his voice is drowning out yours."

Andrea raised his voice and almost shouted, "There's no one here besides us. Your father isn't really here. You're hallucinating him. It's you who bring him here. You can make him leave. Make him leave. You'll see that you have power over him."

She said nothing.

"Do you hear me?"

She nodded.

"Go on then, tell him to go. Tell him out loud, so I can hear."

"Please go, please," she said weakly.

Then she turned to Andrea. "He's not moving. He won't go. He's still here."

"Don't beg him to go. Don't say 'Please.' Order him."

"I don't think I can."

"You can."

She was silent.

"Do it," Andrea said.

"Go away." Her voice was louder than before.

"That isn't loud enough. Shout!"

"Go away! Go away!" she screamed. She almost seemed to lose control of herself.

Then she stopped trembling and looked at Andrea. "He left," she said. "I feel exhausted . . . I can still smell his odor."

"Don't you feel relieved?"

"I'm just too tired."

"That's because you've had a tough struggle. Something has changed now. You've been in the passive victim's role, but now you've established that you're stronger than the apparition. Now you know you can triumph over it."

"My father's smell is gone," she said.

She told me the next day that she had awakened in the morning to see her father sitting at her dressing table, a toothpick in his mouth. She had decided to be bold with him.

"What do you want?" she asked him as she lay in bed. She said it aloud, although she knew he could have known her question without her using her voice.

"You know what I want," he said.

She tried to be strong. "I don't care if you stay here. I'm not going to be bothered."

"I don't care what you say," he replied. "When I leave you, I do so because I want to, not because you tell me to." He started to approach her bed as he said that.

She jumped out of bed, put on a dressing gown, and ran out of the room.

She went downstairs, where she stayed a few hours. Later, when she went upstairs again, the apparition was gone.

She was observing a change in her mood. She was now crying only three or four times a day, which was much less than before. Her appetite had improved, and she was feeling better generally.

At 11:30 on her sixth night at the Centre, she saw her husband Paul, who was there with her, change into her father. The first thing she noticed was that Paul's brown eyes became blue, like her father's. Then his whole face changed into her father's. When she looked away from Paul and back at him, she saw Paul's face again, except his eyes remained blue. As she continued to gaze at him, he started to look like her father once more. Her father was wearing the same clothes as Paul.

It was late to be bothering Andrea and Laura, but she was frightened. She went to their room. Laura was out, but Andrea was there, in bed.

Ruth, Andrea, and Paul told me the next day what ensued.

"Can you come to my room?" Ruth asked Andrea. "I've been seeing Paul turning into my father."

"Yes," he said, and went with her.

She looked at Paul. "He looks gross, just like my father," she told Andrea. "And he has the same disgusting smell that my father had the night he raped me."

She sat on the bed next to Paul, and Andrea sat next to her.

Paul was feeling hopeless. He wanted to do something to help, but when she was seeing him as her father, she just glared at him and shook when he spoke, as if it were her father talking.

Andrea felt she was less frightened than on previous occasions. "Tell your father to go away and stay away," he told her. To Paul he said, "You understand that it's her father I'm telling her to address, though it's you she'll be looking at when she speaks."

"Yes."

"I didn't hear what you said," Ruth commented, "because my father was talking too."

"Why don't you hold Ruth's hand and talk to her?" Andrea said to Paul.

Paul laid his hand on hers. "It's me, Paul—not your father."

She cried and trembled. She felt her hand hurting; it was being held too tightly, and her fingers were being squeezed. She pushed his hand away.

Paul had not been squeezing her hand.

She started to breathe slowly and to concentrate on getting rid of her father. She saw her father's features begin to disappear gradually. Now she saw both Paul and her father instead of just her father. As her father's features faded further, she could see that the man there was Paul. But her father's odor lingered, and the eyes remained blue. "My father's mean old piercing eyes keep glaring at me," she said.

"Look at the eyes more closely," Andrea said, "and say what you see."

She looked. "They're definitely blue." She was much calmer.

They were still blue when Andrea left the room.

Paul and Ruth went on talking. She refused to look at him and told him she didn't want him to sleep in her bed that night, as it would feel like sleeping with her father. She felt he was dirty and didn't even want him to put his arm around her. Yet she knew Paul appealed to her more than any man she had ever known, and told him so. She didn't see how the marriage could last under such circumstances—nor did he. He felt confused and hurt.

He slept on a mattress on the floor at the foot of her bed.

The next morning Ruth and Paul went sight-seeing in London. Whenever Ruth looked at him for more than a few seconds, she saw him change into her father. It always began with the eyes becoming blue. It happened on the subway and in a firearms shop where Paul was explaining something to her about a gun. She "shook off" the experiences, she said, but nonetheless they unnerved her.

After reporting these events in her session with me that day, she told me about an incident from her past.

"My first child, George, was a few months old, old enough to crawl. He and I were visiting my parents. My father was cleaning his guns. I'd kept George near me, but then he crawled around. Suddenly, I heard a shot. A pellet grazed George's face and lodged in the wall. My mind went blank. All I remember is grabbing George and leaving. My mother said I attacked my father and flew all over him, hitting him with my fists. But I have no memory of it. Later my father said it was an accident."

Ruth paused, looked up at me—and gasped. "I see my father now upon your face." She became very, very frightened. She trembled and cried. "I want to leave. I can't stand this."

"I'm not your father," I said. "It's me, Dr. Schatzman. I'm not your father. Your father isn't here. Only you and I are."

"Are you smiling?"

"No."

"Your mouth is smiling."

"No, it isn't."

"Are you sure?"

"Yes. I'm not smiling. I assure you."

She kept staring at me.

"Can I touch your face just to make sure it's yours?"

"Yes."

She touched it and felt my beard. "It's you."

"How could you tell?"

"I felt your beard. My father never has worn one, and his apparition hasn't either."

"You couldn't see my beard?"

"I'm not sure if I was seeing it or not. But I'm sure I felt it."

"How did you feel about touching the face?"

"I was already seeing it mainly as your face before I touched it. I'd be too afraid to touch the apparition's face."

She seemed less frightened than before, and I thought of suggesting something that I realized might strain her trust in my judgment. I decided to risk it.

"I'd like you to try to change me into your father."

She was astonished. "But why?"

"There are a few reasons. Generally, the more one confronts what one fears, the more quickly one becomes unafraid. The more you face the apparition, the less fear you'll have in its company. And if you can make it appear, you'll experience its appearance as being under your control. If you found you could summon it up whenever you wished, you'd probably realize you can send it away whenever you wish."

"Your reasons are good, but I don't like the idea at all. I'll try, though."

Her willingness to try something so seemingly strange after so little encouragement impressed me. Why was she willing? Was she trying to please me by being a cooperative patient? Or was it that she trusted me and believed that following my suggestions would help her? I felt that if in the course of following my proposal she had a fit of panic, it would quickly evaporate without harm to her.[9]

She stared at my face and began to tremble, cry, blush, perspire, and wring her hands. "All right, I'm beginning to see him," she said after about twenty seconds. She looked away from my face.

"Look at me again. Tell me what you see."

"I see small blue eyes, with bushy eyebrows."

My eyes are a nondescript color somewhere between gray, green, and brown; my eyebrows are thin.

"Your complexion has changed," she said, still looking at me. "Your beard has disappeared. You're laughing."

"I'm not."

"I can see your mouth twisted into a smile and can hear laughing."

"I'm not smiling or laughing. Why don't you make him leave now?"

"What?"

"Why don't you make him leave now?"

"I can't hear you above the sound of his laughter."

I shouted, "Why don't you make him leave now!"

"I don't think what you say will make any difference. He's going to stay or come back if *he* wants to." She was still trembling and wringing her hands. "Yet I feel your presence with me, which helps." She continued to look at me. "He's left. I see your face again. The blue eyes were the last thing to change back."

"That was fine. You did well. I think he left because we decided to make him leave. He has his own will only to the extent that you let him have it—which means he doesn't really have it."

"Seeing you turn into my father just then scared me, but not as much as when it happened the first time, without my expecting it. I'm sure glad you changed back to yourself."

The next day she told me, "Last night I dreamed my father was standing near me, saying: 'If Dr. Schatzman's appearance can change so that he looks like me, how do you know I can't look like him? When you think you're seeing him, how do you know it's not me you're seeing?'"

I laughed. "It was clever of you to compose those lines for your father after yesterday's session."

"I composed those lines?"

"It was your dream. Who else could have?"

She looked down at the floor. I thought she might be upset at being held responsible for such a thought.

"I felt so nervous when I awoke," she said. "It would be terrible if what isn't real were real, and if at the end of our relationship you turned into my father and said you'd been him all along."

"How serious are you about that possibility?"

"Not very."

"Good." I felt relieved. I knew I might have been unable to find a convincing argument that I was really the person I appeared to be.

"Are you feeling nervous about trusting me?" I asked.

"I have no one else to trust."

"That might be a reason to be feeling nervous."

She did not reply.

I had an idea for something to do in our session. "Why don't you try to produce the apparition standing or sitting on its own—not on Paul's face, or mine, or anyone's?"

"I'll try, but what's the point?"

"The same as I explained to you yesterday."

She paused for a moment. "All right." She began to tremble, but seemed less frightened than she had the day before, when her father's image had first appeared on my face.

She stared at an empty space in the corner of the room which was opposite her and to my left. "I'm seeing him now. He's wearing a white shirt that's well pressed. He's smiling. I'm not too frightened. I feel I can make him go away."

"I'm sure you can. Could you make him tell you why he's been persecuting you?"

She put her thumb in her mouth and bit it nervously. "I don't need to speak to him since he knows what I'm going to say . . . He's looking at you and laughing . . . He's looking at me and saying 'He's going to need—' and then I can't make out the rest . . . He's saying to me that you can't help me. He's cursing as he's talking . . . I'm still feeling I can do away with him when I want to."

"Fine. Why don't you do it, then?"

She continued to stare at the corner for about ten seconds, and then moved her eyes slowly across the room toward the door to my office.

"He's gone now."

"Good. How are you feeling?"

"Not too bad."

"Can you tell me what you did to bring on the apparition?"

"It's hard to explain. I just concentrated on producing it over there where it appeared." She shifted her position in her chair. "Since I wasn't as frightened this time as I've been before—though I was still nervous—I was able to pay attention to certain details."

"Yes?"

"The colors of the apparition's face were lifelike. Just as in real life, he had gray hairs in his eyebrows. I also noticed that the wall behind where he was standing disappeared from my view, just as it would have if a real person had been standing there."

"How old did he seem to you?"

"His present age. His age when I last saw him about three years ago."

The following day, Ruth announced to me, "I've polished my toenails." She slipped off her sandals to show me. "It's a sign I'm feeling better. I haven't polished them in weeks."

"Good. How do you feel about having another meeting today with you-know-who?"

"I don't want to think about you-know-who . . . Well, all right, if you think it's necessary."

"'Necessary' isn't quite the right word. I think it would be a good idea."

"Shall I do him on his own or on your face?"

"Let's try it on my face again. That seems to have upset you more than doing him on his own."

"I was afraid you'd say that. All right, here goes."

She stared at my face from her seat opposite me.

About half a minute passed. "O.K. Your eyes are blue now, very blue. They're piercing and are staring at me cold and hard. There are red lines in the whites of your eyes."

In fact, my eyes were not inflamed.

"Your forehead has changed. Your nose is wider than usual. Your face isn't shaven, but you don't have a beard. Your complexion is redder. I can't tell if you're smiling or if your lips have parted."

My lips were closed.

"He's smiling now."

I was not smiling. I noted the shift from *"Your* lips" to *"He's* smiling." It suggested that whatever she was looking at was now appearing more like her father than like me.

"He seems delighted to be here," she said.

She was nervous, but far less than on previous occasions.

"What about the clothes?" When she had seen Paul change into her father, the clothes had remained the same ones Paul had actually been wearing.

She studied me. "You have on a red-plaid flannel shirt. I can see it clearly. It has some white stripes, and a little yellow running through it."

I was wearing a solid-color tan shirt underneath a brown jacket with a herringbone design.

"A button is missing on it."

I looked to see if a button was missing from my shirt or jacket—none was.

"The shirt is open at the neck."

My shirt was buttoned at the neck.

"The skin on your neck is suntanned in the shape of a V."

I had no suntan beneath my shirt, nor was I wearing a V-necked undershirt.

Her eyes moved downward. "You're wearing jeans."

I was wearing ordinary trousers.

"I can smell him. It's a soapy smell, as if he just took a bath."

I thought about when I had last bathed. It had not been in the past few hours.

"Could we try something?" she asked.

"Yes."

"Could you get up and walk across the room toward me? I want to see if you take my father along with you as you move, or if you leave him behind sitting in your chair."

"All right." I was pleased with her wish to experiment, and I guessed she knew that.

I got up from my chair and walked across the room to a spot about three feet in front of her and to her right.

Her eyes followed me. "My father moved with you." She looked back at my chair. "Your chair is empty. He didn't stay behind."

I returned to my chair opposite her.

"He moved back to your chair with you . . . I'm feeling frightened by all this."

"There's nothing to be frightened of. You won't be harmed. Relax."

"I can hear you, but your lips aren't moving. Your head—it looks like his head—is moving from side to side as if it's saying no."

I was not shaking my head.

"Could you move toward me again?" she said. "I want to try and leave my father sitting in your chair."

I walked to the same spot I had before.

She continued to stare at my chair. She said, "He's still in your chair . . . He's saying, 'I know what you meant to do. That's why I've stayed in Dr. Schatzman's chair. I've stayed because *I* wanted to.'"

I squatted to take notes.

"He's talking about you, calling you names like 'son of a bitch,' and laughing . . . He says you know about him only what he lets you know, you can never make him go away, he leaves only because he wants to leave, and he'll never stop appearing to me."

I saw that two power struggles were now occurring: the original one between Ruth and the apparition and a newer one between me and the apparition.

"He's saying he's not about to die," Ruth said.

"What does he mean by that?"

"I've sometimes thought his visits were a sign that my actual father would be dying soon. He's saying I'm wrong."

I was still squatting near her chair, taking notes.

"Now he's saying I should look at you."

She did—and caught her breath. She started to tremble again. "He's there, on your face too. There's one of him on your chair and one of him where you are. The one where you are is asking me how I know who's who and is laughing loudly . . . Now he's pretending to write. He's making fun of you. He doesn't have any pen or paper in his hands, but he's playing as if he's writing."

All the time she was saying this, she was staring at me. Apparently, she was not seeing the pen and notebook with which I was actually writing, but was hallucinating their absence. She was seeing only her father's hands making writing movements in the air.

Still looking at me and seemingly hearing her father's words coming from my mouth, she said, "He's saying to me, 'I'm stronger than Dr. Schatzman. Your telling him about the fucking rape doesn't change anything.' He's laughing . . . 'Tell him the whole story, and he'll make you right.' He's saying it mockingly . . . It's as if my father is here now, saying he's not ashamed of having raped me . . . I'm feeling ill." She was very upset, trembling and breathing hard.

"Can I touch your hand?" I asked.

"Yes."

Gently I rested my hand on the back of her hand, which was gripping the arm of the chair.

"It's his hand. It's big and fat, and its skin is rough. You're squeezing my hand too hard."

My hand is not big, fat, or rough, and was not squeezing her hand at all.

"When you're near me, I can really smell him."

"I think we've had enough of him for today. Let's get rid of him." My hand was still resting on hers.

She looked at my chair. "He's going, but he's laughing . . . He's saying he's going because he wants to go. He's laughing very hard." Her eyes moved to her left, away from me and toward the office door. "He's gone."

"Look at me, and tell me what you see." I was still crouching to her right.

"I'm afraid to."

"Come on."

She looked at me. "It's you."

I moved back to my chair and sat down.

She said, "I feel queasy in my stomach and nauseous when he's around. This meeting took a lot out of me. I feel tired, as if I'd been working all day."

"You did well. You illustrated once again that you can get rid of him when you want to—despite what he says—and that he doesn't harm you. The worst he accomplished is to tire you."

"I guess so. When he appears on your face, he can't harm *you,* can he?"

I laughed. "I don't see how—but thanks for your concern."

"If I thought he could harm you, I'd end my therapy now," she said, apparently unaware of my irony. "If he hurt anyone, I'd rather it were me than someone else."

"I'm not worried about his harming me. He doesn't affect me. When you're seeing me as him, my experience of myself is the same as it ordinarily is. Only your experience of me is changed. You needn't worry about his harming you either. By the way, does your father own a red-plaid flannel shirt like the one you described?"

"I don't know."

"Does Paul have one?"

"No. I know he doesn't."

That night Ruth dreamed that her father appeared to her. She told me the dream the next day.

"In the dream my father was bare-chested. He said to me, 'Don't you set foot in my house again.' I asked him, 'Why?' He replied, 'You should tell Dr. Schatzman that if he has as much sense as you give him credit for, he'll warn you that I can do lots of damage to you—even if you're not wise enough to know that yourself.' I said, 'You can't hurt me.'"

She was trembling a little now.

"What do you think your father was threatening you about?" I asked.

"I don't know. His warning me not to set foot in his house could be his getting even for our asking him to go yesterday."

"Could be. He acted in the dream as a real person who was feeling rejected might have. But I believe he's no more real than any dream figure is. Was there more in the dream?"

"Yes. He said, 'You need a priest—not Dr. Schatzman—as you don't have much time.' I guess he was hinting that I'll be dying soon." She was continuing to tremble. "He said, 'You shouldn't trust your doctor. If you want to play the games he wants to play, you'll have to pay.' I don't know what he means by 'games.' I've been holding onto you and everything you say as a life jacket. He's trying to shatter my confidence in you. Then he said, 'You forgot to tell the doctor you'd cut your hair. If you tell him that, he'll see how deranged you were.'

"During his raping me, when he had his orgasm, his semen wet my face and got into my hair. I had long hair then, so long that I could sit on it." She began to cry. "After he'd finished, I went to the sink to wash my hair. I kept trying to wash that stuff out. I thought it would never come out. I took up my mother's sewing scissors and cut off some of my hair." Ruth was crying bitterly as she talked. "Everyone told me I'd done a crazy thing cutting off my own hair. At that moment I had probably been deranged, because I'd thought I'd never be able to wash the semen out—though I didn't know it was semen.

"My father had the nerve to take the hair I'd cut off and braid it—three long strands. And he put the braid in the family Bible as a bookmark!"

"How bizarre!" I said softly.

She nodded in agreement. "It's still there! It's like a trophy for him, like a scalp for an Indian warrior."

I wondered what his using her hair as a bookmark for a Bible implied. It could indicate the utmost contempt for her feelings and for whatever the Bible meant to him. Probably his attack upon her meant something very different to him than it did to her—or to me.

"You say you were deranged for having cut off your hair. But what about your father's behavior in having assaulted you in the first place, and doing what he did with your hair?"

"Yes, I guess he was a bit off himself."

"A bit off" seemed a sizable understatement.

"I'm so afraid of him. I just can't deal with all this as my imagination. I was terrified of coming here to see you today. I thought my life would be endangered. But my need to come was greater than my terror. I desperately need your help."

"You're getting my help. Why the terror?"

"I'm not sure. Probably it's due to the dream. When he said I'd forgotten to tell you about cutting my hair, I felt he didn't fear my telling you anything. That meant you were no threat to him."

"If I were no threat to him, he wouldn't be bothering to tell you not to trust me."

"You've got a point." She had stopped crying.

"Had you forgotten only to tell me about the hair cutting, or had you forgotten it had happened?"

"This is my first memory of it for many years. Some time after the rape—I don't know when—I'd stopped being aware of it."

She might have kept the incident out of awareness for so long owing to the distress originally associated with it. Why then had she not forgotten her father's assault altogether? Perhaps because, though the assault had been painful, it had not been of her own doing. But she had cut her own hair off, and had been considered crazy for doing it. Even now, she thought she had been deranged. Why had she recalled the hair cutting at this time? Maybe she had initially suppressed her memory of that behavior because it had been labeled crazy, and maybe all the reassurance she had been recently receiving from me that she was not crazy had given her the courage to remember it. I found the way the occurrence returned to her—in a dream and from her father's lips—fascinating.

*　　*　　*

The next day, her eleventh at the Crisis Centre, was her last day there. Paul's leave from work was ending and she was needed at home. Her state of mind had been progressively improving, and I was not apprehensive about her leaving the Centre, despite the apparition's continuing harassment of her. She, however, felt uneasy.

"I'm worried about coping at home," she told me. "I'm afraid of having bad dreams and apparitions in my bedroom. They're more of an invasion there than elsewhere. My children are going to be depending on me. I don't know if I'm ready. I want to be happy and to make people around me happy. I'm glad to be going home, but I'm terribly afraid too."

"How are you feeling about going back to Paul?"

"I dread what could happen if he tries to have sex with me. But I'm also frightened he might not. I hope he hasn't lost interest. He's probably fed up with me, and I don't blame him."

Paul came to the Centre that last day to spend some time with her before driving her home. The children remained at home with a family friend.

I decided to spend a few hours at the Centre to give Ruth extra support.

Ruth chatted with Paul for about half an hour.

Afterward she confided in me, "When I saw Paul, my stomach was tied in knots, and my conversation was strained."

I had misgivings about her remark. She seemed to feel more relaxed with me than with him, but it was to him that she would now be returning.

Ruth, Paul, Andrea, Laura, and I gathered together in the Centre's living room for the last meeting before Ruth and Paul's departure.

Paul seemed troubled. He looked at me. "What course do you think Ruth's illness, or condition, or whatever you call it, is likely to take?"

The way he phrased his question seemed opportune. "I can't

say with certainty," I said, "as I've never known or heard about anyone in just her situation before. But she's been making progress, and I think she's likely to continue to."

"I'm pleased she didn't end up going to a mental hospital," he said.

I was finding it slightly odd for us to be talking about Ruth as if she was not in the room. However, since the conversation seemed useful, I was prepared to go on with it. I looked at her to let her know I was aware of her presence.

"I have another question," Paul said. "What should I do if she starts seeing her father's face on my face?"

"Has she told you how I coped when she saw him on my face?"

"Yes. I was relieved to hear she'd seen him on someone's face besides mine." He smiled a bit wryly.

"Since you know what method I used, you might try the same thing," I said.

What else could I say? I was aware my answer was not satisfactory, but I could think of none that would be.

There was a moment of silence. Then Ruth asked me, "Do you think I'm crazy for seeing an apparition?"

Why did she still want reassurance on this issue? Perhaps she thought Paul needed to hear she was sane, though I believed she was really the one who needed to hear it.

"Most of the problems for which you first came to see me and to stay with Laura and Andrea have been clearing up," I said. "Suppose all your original complaints disappeared completely, but you went on seeing the apparition. Suppose it only manifested when you summoned it and vanished whenever you wished. And suppose finally it stopped menacing and threatening you. That's where the course you're now on seems to be leading."

In offering this opinion, I knew that I was increasing the likelihood of such an outcome.

"Could your experience of the apparition be labeled then as crazy?" I said. "As sick? As a symptom? It would be more justified to see you as having a capacity or a talent that other people are lacking. That's how I think of you. Whether you'd regard yourself as mad or as gifted could greatly affect your self-esteem and your moods. You'd feel better about yourself if you saw yourself as having a skill, not as being ill."

Ruth and Paul gave no response. Fleetingly I wondered if they thought me crazy for saying that.

I went on, looking at Ruth. "You remember the Senoi, after conquering their dream enemies, make them give gifts. The Senoi also make servants or allies out of their dream antagonists to help them deal with future dream difficulties. So far, you've been trying to render your father's apparition less intimidating. Perhaps eventually you could find some way to benefit from your experience of him. Maybe you could ask favors of him or enlist his help."

She laughed. "If I could get him to do what I wanted, the first thing I'd do would be to give you a taste of your own medicine by sending him to you."

Everyone laughed.

Ruth's Past

SINCE meeting Ruth, I had been noting the facts of her life as they came up in her conversation. Eventually my picture of her past became fairly extensive, and I present it here.

One generally samples and gathers past events in the light of their apparent relevance to one's present concerns. In doing so, one lets the facts adapt themselves to the order which one now gives them. And one continually preserves the possibility of changing the meanings of each fact. Though nothing can be added to the content of the past—one's own or anyone else's—and nothing can be removed from it, there is a sense in which we create our pasts, or at least create their meanings. That is why all biographies, including clinical ones, are, to some degree, works of imagination.

"My mother was born in California," Ruth said, "and is a housewife. My father was born in Oregon and is a carpenter. The marriage was the first one for both of them. Besides my younger sister, Jane, I have a sister, Mallory, five and a half years older than me, and a brother, Andrew, four years older. I was born in 1951 in a hospital near my parents' home. My mother was thirty when I was born, and my father was thirty-five.

"Both my mother and grandmother say that I was a month and a half premature, becuase my mother fell while carrying water from a well. They told me I weighed three and a half or four pounds at birth, that my crying sounded 'cheepy,' that I had to be kept in the hospital longer than usual, and that I was so small they took me home in a shoe box. That all sounds to me like I was premature. But I've seen my birth certificate, which says the pregnancy lasted nine months and doesn't give any birth weight. I've asked my mother about it, but she's never explained.

"My father's name is on my birth certificate, but he told me once when he was drunk that he's not my real father. Whenever I've asked my mother about it, she's denied it—and has burst into tears. My father disappeared for long periods of time, and my mother had men friends. But I look like my father and I believe he's my real father. Maybe he wished he wasn't my father, so his sexual interest in me would seem less wrong.

"When I was six weeks old, he left us and used a different name. He had forged checks and wanted to escape arrest. Eventually he was found, arrested, and convicted, and spent five years in jail. He came back home when I was seven.

"He was often in jail afterward for short times, usually for getting drunk and disturbing the peace or something.

"A few times he was a mental patient, both before I was born and after he came back to the family. A doctor called him schizophrenic.[10] Once, I was home for a weekend from the children's institution, and photographs of my sister Mallory, who'd just won a beauty contest, were all over the house. My father turned them all facedown; he thought they were laughing at him. 'What's going on?' I asked my mother. All she said was, "Ssh-h-h." Soon afterward my mother had him put in a mental hospital.

"Some of his mental hospitalizations were due to his drinking.

He used drugs, too, and I think he was an addict. I can remember him injecting himself with paregoric.

"When I think about my beginnings, I wonder how I ever managed to turn out as I have—not that I'm such a marvelous person, but I'm not a criminal or a drunk.

"Mallory as a teenager, like me at a younger age, was always being accused by my father of having sexual relations with boys. She never did. She got married when she was seventeen, and since then she's had two nervous breakdowns. I don't know much about them. I believe they were because of her marriage. My brother, Andrew, was a juvenile delinquent. Now he's an electrician, and married with three children.

"I think my relationship with my grandma—my mother's mother—saved me. After I came home from the hospital where I was born, I lived with my mother and grandmother and was closer to my grandmother than to anyone else. When I was a child, my grandma was my world.

"My mother sent me, Mallory, and Andrew to a children's home when I was three years old. I can remember that day. I was riding in a car. Mallory and my Uncle Herman were in the front seat. Some woman I didn't know, who I later found out was a social worker, was driving. My brother, my grandmother, and I were in the back. My grandma had me on her lap. She was crying. There were mountains on either side of us, and I was hoping we could hurry through them just in case they decided to collapse.

"The car finally stopped at a house with lots of children. We got out of the car. When we started to run up the walk, the backs of my knees hurt. I stopped. Something wasn't right. A lady walked over to us. She appeared to be ten feet tall and had ugly hair and eyes. She didn't seem to think too highly of me. Well, I would just stay close to Grandma. The big lady spoke sharply to Andrew, and I knew he was about to cry. Mallory and Grandma didn't look happy either. I announced I was ready to go home. I was expecting to spend that night with Grandma. The lady looked down at me and said, 'You have a new home now with me.' My grandmother started to cry, and this big lady took me from her. I was scared. I started to fight and cry. The lady shook me and slapped my face. She said I was spoiled, and she had never had a child fight her like that before. Why was she taking me away from Grandma? Grandma needed me; she had told me so every night. Who would sleep with her? And who would keep me warm at night? My arms hurt from the big lady holding me so tight. Now the car was leaving. Inside it I saw my Uncle Herman holding my grandmother. This all had to be a mistake. I thought this was my punishment for once having thrown sand in a girl's hair. I was so sorry; I would never do it again.

"The next treat in store for me was for that big lady to cut off all my hair. Grandma had always liked my long hair. She had spent an hour that morning making it all pretty. Grandma would really be mad. How I hated that lady!

"That big lady, I found out, was the housemother. The children used to call her Big Mama.

"This was the same institution I later lived in after my father attacked me. Even in my teens, I was still angry at Big Mama. When Big Mama would say 'good morning' to me I'd tell her, 'Go to hell.' I was fourteen when she died, and I was pleased at her death. 'Good, now she can't beat anyone anymore,' I said, and I wouldn't go to the funeral.

"When I was first there, at three, Grandma had wanted to keep me at home, thinking I was too young to be sent away. But my mother wanted to start a new life away from Grandma and from the responsibility of looking after us children. She thought my grandma was too old to look after me on her own, and she wanted us children to be together.

"I don't like to think about my mother putting us away, but I wonder what the new life was that she began. I know she moved to the town the children's home was in, and got an evening job there as a telephone operator. The town was a few hundred miles from where we'd been living and where Grandma went on living. Occasionally we'd see our mother.

"I took a long time to get used to being away from Grandma. At night I cried about being separated from her—though when children at the home cried, they were told not to feel sorry for themselves. I pushed away anyone who tried to hug me. I also stopped eating. I had to go to a hospital. Then Grandma started visiting me with gifts. And in the summer and for Christmas, I visited her, and we'd sleep together again.

"I stayed at the children's home for almost two years and hated it the whole time. When I was five, my mother took the three of us back to live with her in a two-bedroom apartment. Grandma sometimes came and took me to stay with her.

"At seven, I saw my father. One day my mother sent me to the store to get some bread. On the way back I saw a man looking at houses on the street. At first I thought he might have been one of my mother's brothers, but when I got closer I saw he was my father. I don't know how I knew who he was. He didn't recognize me. He asked me if I knew where Mrs. Sergeant (my mother) lived. I answered yes, that I was going there and would take him with me.

"Later, we were in the house, and he or my mother asked me if I knew who he was. I said, yes, he was my daddy. I was happy. I wanted him to come outside with me so I could show everyone what a good daddy I had. He wasn't as pretty as I'd hoped, but he would do just fine.

"At that time he'd just been paroled from prison. He lived with us a short time before leaving, but promised to come back soon for good. I was about as happy as I'd ever been, and couldn't wait to have my own father with me and with my brother and sister.

"The next important stage in my life was my father's return. However, he wasn't there very long before what had seemed a blessing turned out to be a living hell. He was mean, especially when he drank, and he drank often. Once, he jumped on us all. Andrew, who was about twelve, fought back. My father smashed him against a shelf, breaking his head open.

"He was particularly mean and violent to me. I used to feel responsible for his meanness and his drinking, as if they were my fault. I couldn't understand what I had done wrong that had led to all this happening.

"When my father would come into a room I was in, I'd be frightened. I never understood why. Maybe it was how he looked at me. In his presence, I somehow felt something dreadful would happen to me. That feeling turned out to be as true as any feeling I've ever had. To this day, he still looks funny at me.

"And yet there were times he could be such a good father, as good as Paul is, or as you must be. When I was eight, which was right in the middle of the period of his meanness to me, I was sick once with flu. I was so sick I couldn't go upstairs without passing out. He made a bed for me on the couch. He sat next to me for two days, putting cold rags on me and giving me medicine. I'd awaken in the middle of the night, and he'd still be sitting there. And I wasn't afraid of him. He'd say, 'You'll be all right, baby. I won't leave you.'

"Memories like that make me feel guilty about my bad feelings toward him. I can see now how confused I must have been. I wonder how a child of that age can cope with all I had to cope with.

"While my father and I were living in the same house, if he wanted me to do something, he'd get down one of his guns from its place on the wall and threaten to shoot me. It scared me to death. I'm still uneasy about guns.

"Near the time of the rape, before I left home, he once shot at me and missed. He'd been drinking. He came after me with a gun, saying I was the goddamned bastard who had been fucking in the playground. The shot blew a big hole in the wall near my head. He reloaded the gun and came after me again. I ran to the house of a woman neighbor and hid there. She phoned the police, who came to the house and took him away. He was cursing me as they took him away. They kept him in jail for a few weeks.

"My mother recently told me something I'd forgotten: five pieces of buckshot had landed in the side of my head and had later been removed, and I'd been deaf in that ear for a week.

"When he shot at me, my mother was scared. She didn't say anything to him then, because you couldn't talk to him when he was drunk. She threatened him later that she'd leave him unless he straightened up. But she'd said that so many times that we got worn out from hearing it."

The father's alleged reason for shooting at Ruth—that she "had been fucking in the playground"—intrigued me. Was he angry with her because he believed she had been behaving immorally? If so, what did he think was immoral? Her having sexual relations, or her having them with someone other than him? Probably he was jealous—morbidly jealous—of imagined sexual behavior on her part. Morbid sexual jealousy is usually directed toward a spouse, not a ten-year-old offspring.

"Years later he took a shot at my son George. He wasn't drinking that time, but he always said that the incident was an accident.

"Many times after a long drinking bout, my father hallucinated. He cried and pleaded with people to buy him more whiskey to get relief from the hallucinations, and sometimes I did. At times he'd hallucinate in jail after getting arrested for being drunk. One of those times he thought a pack of dogs were barking at him, and he saw moss growing on the walls of his cell. He'd see bugs and snakes too. The animals he saw sometimes bit him. He felt the bites and saw his wounds bleeding. After coming out of this state, he'd recognize that he'd hallucinated the animals, the bites, and the blood.

"A doctor told us that these hallucinations, which occurred when he withdrew from alcohol, were symptoms of delirium tremens or DTs. I've never had that sort of hallucination.

"One time in my childhood, I can't remember when, he was in jail—I think he was there for drunken driving or disturbing the peace—and he slashed his wrists. He was found lying in a pool of blood, and was rushed to the hospital. While my mother and I were standing next to his hospital bed, he told us he'd tried to kill himself because he'd thought a mob of people were outside the jail wanting to lynch him for something he'd done to me. He'd heard them talking about him. 'That's terrible, let's lynch him,' he'd heard someone say. He decided not to allow them the pleasure of hanging him. My mother asked him what they supposed he'd done to me. 'Damned if I know,' he said. I think the voices of the mob of people talking about him were probably hallucinations."

"Did your father," I asked Ruth, "ever hallucinate when he hadn't been drinking?"

"I don't know—but there's a lot about him I don't know."

I knew that the father's experiences and behavior just described are typical of some individuals after an intense drinking bout. They feel apprehensive and fearful, hear voices which commonly accuse them of wrongdoing or which threaten attack, and are likely to attempt suicide. Afterward, they can recall vividly the events, feelings, and thoughts that were happening. This condition is called acute alcoholic hallucinosis. Some of these persons go on in time to act in such ways that they are labeled schizophrenic.

"That time when my father tried suicide, he almost died before my mother and I got to the hospital. The nurse told my mother that the doctor had thought he was already dead." The doctor had told the nurse, 'Leave him; cover him up with a sheet.' But the nurse wasn't so sure; she thought she'd seen him move. She called to him, 'Mr. Sergeant, if you can hear me, wiggle your thumb.' She believed she saw him wiggle it, and she went to get the doctor. The doctor came and pounded on his chest. My father later said he'd heard them discussing whether or not he was alive, but he'd felt helpless. He'd been aware of the nurse running out of the room, and then of the doctor thumping on his chest. After he'd been found to be alive, he was rushed to the operating room for surgery of some sort—on his heart, I think."

It occurred to me that the father's return from the dead could have strikingly impressed Ruth as a girl and made her believe he had superhuman powers. Such a belief could have intensified her fear of his apparition later on.

"Were there any teachings about death or religion in your upbringing?" I asked Ruth.

"My father and grandmother were Catholic, and the children's home was Methodist. I was brought up to believe that after you die, you lie in the ground and your soul stays with your body, until

Judgement Day. Then Christ, or God, or whoever's responsible gathers up all souls, and you're measured for your good deeds and sins, and sent to heaven or hell."

"Do you still believe that?"

"I don't think so."

Ruth told me that religion wasn't very important to her.

"After my mother had decided that my father and I couldn't live in the same house, I went to live first with my friend Becky. I'd met Becky, who's about my age, soon after leaving the children's home the first time. We've been friends ever since. Becky has probably been as important to me as my grandmother, in a different way. While I was at Becky's house—I was eleven—her older brother, Carl, who was twelve or thirteen, was there. My father accused me of screwing him, which I hadn't. Eventually I had to leave that house.

"My mother and I then visited a probate judge at a courthouse. The judge asked me if I understood what was happening and if I wanted to go to the children's home. Yes, I replied, the children's home was a nice place and I knew some girls from school there. I guess I felt I had no choice in the matter. My mother cried and said she'd get me out of there when school was out, nine months later.

"That nine months got stretched out a lot—I stayed in the children's home for nearly seven years and never lived with my parents again.

"This time I arrived at the institution on my own in a taxi. Already I hated the place more than when I'd left it. I was assigned to a cottage of ten girls. I had to undergo all the usual tests and fights before being accepted by them.

"My best friend was a diary to whom I told everything. It was stolen before I left, but it had served its purpose.

"During this stay in the children's home, I visited my family once a month—that was all the supervisors at the institution allowed me.

"When I went home to my parents, my father would be there.

He and I generally wouldn't say anything to each other. If he was drunk, I'd get frightened and leave.

"Once, he visited the institution when he was drunk. He tried to run me down in his car and drove it onto the lawn. Also, he tried to get into my cottage, which wasn't allowed.

"The police were called. When they came, he tried to fight them. They beat him with clubs until his head bled and he was knocked unconscious. I felt as if it were my fault. I felt on his side when they were beating him, but I couldn't do anything.

"He was arrested and went to jail. The doctor and I tried to visit him, but the police wouldn't let us in. I wanted to press charges against the police, but my mother told me not to."

I thought that the person the father was revealed to be suggested that his apparition was a facsimile of the real man, in behavior as well as in appearance.

I asked Ruth early in her stay at the Crisis Centre, "How are you feeling toward your actual father?"

"I wouldn't go near him," she said, "even onto the same street he's on.

"I feel a sickening hatred toward him. I've been hoping he'll die soon. If I were face to face with him, I'd try to kill him. Why shouldn't I? In killing my childhood world, he killed me.

"Yet there's a strong feeling between him and me. In a way I'm closer to him than to anyone else in the world. I find it hard to explain the feeling. It's not a closeness in the sense that we confide in one another. It's that there's so much going on emotionally between us."

How similar, I thought, was her attitude toward his apparition: she had been unwilling to enter a public place for fear of meeting up with it. She had been wishing to kill it off. And a lot had been going on emotionally between her and it.

The history shows that however perverse the father's behavior toward Ruth, he was deeply interested in her; his perverse behavior was a way of expressing his interest. The father's apparition was also interested in her—and also expressed it most bizarrely. The father's interest, though oddly displayed, was apparently more than she got from her mother.

Ruth and I were to gain a new viewpoint about the father's leaving the family after her birth, about the rape, about other of his actions, and about his thinking. But to disclose now the means we were to use in doing so would be premature, as we had not yet discovered the means ourselves.

"When I was thirteen and living at the children's home, I started to date Paul, who was my classmate. He and I went together from then on.

"His family always disapproved of me, because I was living at the children's home. They were planning to send him away to military school when he finished high school, to get him away from me for four years. They said that if after four years of separation we still loved each other, we could marry. In our last year of high school—I'd been accepted at college—he said to me, 'Marry me now or never.' We got married secretly in February and told our parents at our graduation four months later. So I didn't go to college after all; I got a job instead.

"We first went to bed together a few months before our marriage. I was sixteen. Suddenly, after we first did it, I started to detest my long hair though Paul liked it long. He pleaded with me not to cut it off. I insisted. I went to the beauty parlor and got a pixie haircut. At the time, I didn't link what I was doing with cutting off my hair after the rape—I'd forgotten all about that.

"At the start, our sexual relationship was awful. I was so tight, it was hard for him to get inside me, and he felt pain. I felt pain too, and I bled. I saw a gynecologist about it who was no help.

"It was about two years before I could enjoy sex. Even then I didn't enjoy it much, and went on feeling pain, though eventually I was able to climax. I'd get up and shower to wash away the blood. Sometimes there was enough bleeding to make me think I was having a period. I thought intercourse was disturbing my internal organs. I'd go to doctors and tell them, but they couldn't find anything.

"I know my sexual troubles had to do with hang-ups about the rape and my father. Before I was old enough to know what sex was, he had already made it ugly for me.

"Despite these sexual problems, I've generally been satisfied with my marriage. My only complaint—and it's not a big one—is that I feel more dependent on Paul than I'd like. I allow him to make decisions for me which I know I'm capable of making for myself."

There was a type of event, different from what I have just been relating, which Ruth thought was important to tell me. From time to time, breaking into her life—and her forebears' lives—were occurrences of a special sort: visits from apparitions.

Perhaps the apparitions' entry into her forebears' lives had made it likely that they would enter hers. Whether such experiences ordinarily run in families I do not know.

"Grandma used to tell me a tale about something that happened long ago. When she was a girl, about nine years old, her parents bought a house. Grandma shared a bedroom in this house with her sister, who was two years older. The two girls began to complain of hearing a baby·crying at night. Their mother would come into their room and say it was probably a cat they were hearing. The girls continued to hear the crying, night after night. After the family had lived there for a while, a woman in the same town told the family that she'd once lived in that house. She'd given birth to a dead baby in the same room that Grandma and her sister were now sleeping in. Because of that awful experience the woman had moved away, and sold the house to the people from whom Grandma's parents later bought it. After hearing that story, Grandma wouldn't sleep in the room."

From the grandmother's age I calculated the crying sounds she had heard probably occurred about 1890. Between then and the time Ruth was old enough to have understood the tale at least

sixty years elapsed. During those sixty-odd years, the grandmother's memory of the experience might have changed. In telling
and retelling the story, she could have unwittingly begun to falsify
it to heighten its dramatic effect. It was impossible to find out now
whether a cat had made the crying sounds. However, the fact of
the grandmother's telling Ruth this story implied that the
grandmother believed, or at least seriously entertained the possibility, that someone's spirit or ghost can make its presence
known to living people. She had probably conveyed her viewpoint
to Ruth.

In Ruth's father's background a certain remarkable event had
happened—or was alleged to have happened.

"Years ago my father had had a sister, Debbie, a year or two
younger than him, who died at seventeen. Debbie had been a
heroin addict and became a prostitute to support her habit.
Debbie's mother had thrown her out of the house and forbidden
her to return. One morning, Debbie's mother and two of Debbie's
brothers—one of them was my father—were sitting on their porch
at home when they saw a horse and carriage draw up on the street
in front of the house. Debbie got out, walked to the wooden front
gate, and stood there without opening it. She looked ill, as if she
needed some heroin. She walked down the street and disappeared.

"'I told her not to come back here,' Debbie's mother said to the
brothers.

"Just as Debbie disappeared from view, a policeman came up
the street to say Debbie had just died in a hospital of an overdose.

"That was impossible, the mother said, since they'd just seen
her.

"They could not have seen her, the policeman said, because her
body was at the morgue.

"The mother and two brothers went to the morgue where they
identified Debbie's body."

I had heard many stories of a person's apparition manifesting at
just the time or very near the time of that person's death.[12] The
observer or observers of the apparition often, though not always,
were near and dear to the deceased person. Several observers may

collectively have seen the apparition at the same time and place. And material appurtenances, such as a walking stick, a cigar, or—as in this incident—a horse and carriage, sometimes have manifested together with the apparition. I reckoned that this event occurred about 1930. Debbie's mother had told this story to Ruth's mother, who had told it to Ruth. Ruth's father had told Ruth the same story.

I knew that only by speaking to the alleged witnesses could I evaluate the authenticity of the anecdote. My interest in the tale, as in the previous one, was in noting that Ruth's family had let phenomena penetrate its boundaries that do not gain entry into many people's worlds.

"At the children's home, shortly before my fourth birthday, I saw my first apparition—or the first one I recall seeing. Later, I saw the same apparition four more times, three nights in a row when I was nine, and once again at sixteen. Each time it frightened me, which shows that I was afraid of apparitions long before being visited by my father's apparition.

"At six or seven, I woke in the night once to see a figure in my room which I thought was real, but which the person I was with didn't see. I was visiting my grandmother. Up the street from her a crazy lady was living. We had to go by her house every day to get to the store to buy our candy. Her hair would be way out and frizzled-looking as if it had never been brushed. She wasn't old—I'd been told she was in her thirties—but she looked a lot older. They had her in a big yard with a chain fence so that she couldn't get out and hurt people. Sometimes they'd have to chain her when her mother was going to feed her because she'd be violent to her mother. The mother couldn't go out in the yard unless her husband was with her. The lady would shit in the yard and throw it at you if you got too close. When we would walk by the house, she'd run to the fence and try to climb over it. My brother, sister, and I, and a big black girl who would go with us, used to pick up scrap metal to take to the stores to sell. Usually on the way back, the older children would torment me by grabbing me and saying they were going to throw me over the fence and put me in with her. Meanwhile she'd be trying to climb the fence and she'd be shaking it. I thought she was so strong she could pull a tree up out of the ground.

"One particular day, this big black girl had bought herself an ice-cream cone. As my brother, my sister, that black girl, and I went by, they grabbed me by the back of the dress. They made like they were going to throw me inside the fence with the lady. The lady terrified me and she was screaming. She couldn't talk. She was making all these awful sounds. You could hardly see her face for her hair.

"At one point she picked up some shit and threw it across the fence at us. Eventually, we got past her with the black girl asking her if she wanted a bite of the ice-cream cone. We got home, and then I guess I'd forgotten about it for the rest of the day.

"That night I dreamed about her. I was in Grandma's bed. It was a great big bed, with lots and lots of blankets on it. I dreamed this crazy lady was in our house walking around in Grandma's room, looking for that ice-cream cone. I woke up, and I could still see the lady in the room. I started crying and woke up Grandma. She didn't see anyone. She immediately jumped out and got the light on, and when she did, the crazy lady was gone. Grandma wrapped around me a crocheted blanket she'd made and held me in her lap for a long time. She told me the crazy lady was asleep in her own bed in her own house and wasn't in the room, and if I liked we could go down and see her. I didn't want to go. I wanted to stay in bed. Grandma checked the lock on the door and went through all the rooms in the house to make sure for me there was no one there. I wanted her to get back in bed, and for us to get under the covers.

"The next morning after breakfast we walked down to this lady's house, and her mother came outside. Grandma told the mother about my dream, and she asked had the lady been in her own bed that night, or had she been out wandering around the neighborhood. Her mother told us she'd been in her own bed. She told me not to be afraid of her, that she couldn't get out. I was pleased she was going to stay inside the fence. Grandma told me there was no way the lady could hurt me—the lady had been in bed, what I had seen was a dream, and I wasn't to be afraid of it. She said she would always get up with me, and look and see what was there, and if I wasn't with her, I should get up myself and look. Finally I felt reassured.

"Once, at the children's home, before I was four, I awoke from a bad dream about Grandma. The dream made me know even more that I had to get to her. I sat up in my bed, which was a baby's bed with bars or side rails around it. A man was standing at the foot of my bed. I could see the upper part of his body, but my bed blocked his legs. He was tall and thin, and his hair was light. He had on a white top, like a doctor's top, with a button by the collar on one side. He just stood there, not moving, not speaking. He didn't look mean. His face had a sweet expression, almost smiling. I didn't know who he was or what he was doing there. He wasn't supposed to be in the room. I thought he might hurt me.

"I cried and screamed, until all the other little girls were awake. He just stood there smiling. It seemed like ages before anyone came to my rescue. It was lucky it wasn't a fire. Finally Big Mama arrived. She turned on the light, and he disappeared. It was as if he were hiding from Big Mama, not wanting her to see him. That frightened me more. I'm sure I didn't know what a ghost was. To me he was a real man. I took one look at Big Mama and knew she was furious. I'd woken her up, and there was nothing to show her. I started to tell her about the man. She said I'd been dreaming. I knew I hadn't. I felt his presence, even with the light on. I knew that the moment she turned the light out and left the room, I'd see him again. Each time she'd head for the light, I'd get up and throw my leg over the bar of the bed to go with her. She was all I had to hold on to, and I was going with her whether she liked it or not. She could have beaten me, and I still couldn't have stayed in that room without her. She didn't want to let me go to her bed, but eventually she said, 'I guess if I'm going to get any sleep tonight, you're going to have to come with me.' I swallowed my pride and went with her. I spent the rest of the night lying awake in bed with her, with the light on, wondering who the man was.

"At nine years old, I saw him again. One night at home I fell asleep with the hall light on. It was still on when I awoke. There he was, dressed the same way, the same expression on his face. As before, he was standing at the foot of my bed, not moving. I cried out. From the next room my mother shouted to me to shut up. I begged and begged her to come, and finally she did. She turned on the light in my room. She said I'd had a bad dream. I said it wasn't a dream, and I'd seen the man before, wearing the same white shirt that looked like a doctor's shirt. She told me to be quiet, there was no man there, that was a silly idea, and I should go back to sleep and not call her anymore. She turned my bedroom light out and went back to her bed, but I was still afraid to look at the foot of my bed.

"The next night it happened again. At first, my mother was furious with me. My daddy told her not to go to me, and he yelled at me to shut up. I told her to come to me as fast as she could. My daddy and she came to my room together. He turned on the light and told me to lay my ass down and go back to sleep. My mother was more puzzled about it than she'd been the first night, and more understanding than my daddy. After they left, I laid my face on the pillow and wouldn't look up.

"Before I went to bed the third night my mother gave me mineral oil to help me sleep. It was her 'cure-all'; she'd give it to us for stomachache, and pour it into our ears for earache. I lay awake a long time, afraid to go to sleep. I did fall asleep, and then awoke. There he was. I wasn't surprised, since I knew he'd be there. This time I made sure that I was awake and sitting up. I called out to my mother that I was awake and seeing him. Daddy called out, 'Oh, shit!' They told me to come to them, but I was afraid to move out of my bed. All the time the man didn't get angry or aggressive, or even frown. I pleaded with my mother to come quickly. I heard her say to my daddy, 'I'll go,' which I was thankful for. She turned on my light, and the man was gone. 'Is there a man standing there?' she asked me. She made me look under my bed and in all the closets. She asked me what he looked like. I told her. He was clean-shaven. His face was long. His nose was straight and pointed. His teeth were even and pretty. He had one hand on my bed and the other at his side. She asked if I'd ever seen him before in reality, if he was someone I knew. I said I didn't think so. She asked me if he'd said anything. I said, 'No.' She wasn't angry or aggravated that I'd gotten her up. I said I wanted Grandma, who lived in a different town. She told me Grandma would be coming soon.

"At sixteen, when I was in the children's home again, I saw him once more. I was sleeping in a room with three beds, in the bed nearest the door. That way I could be near the light in the hall. I woke, and my old friend was standing at the foot of my bed, slightly to my right, without moving, just as he had each previous time. I can't think of any way in which he looked or acted differently this time than he had before. I sat up. I didn't call to anyone at first. Oh, no, I thought, now I'll be afraid to go to sleep. I wasn't afraid, though, the way I'd been before, I called to one of the other two girls in the room. She didn't wake up or even move, and I got frightened. I called Mrs. King, my housemother, which woke the two girls. Mrs. King put on the light. I told her I'd seen a man standing at the foot of my bed, and as a child I'd seen him standing in the same place. She seemed to understand. At least she didn't fuss at me. 'Maybe he's your future husband,' she said, 'your Prince Charming to take you away—and you've scared him off.' She said if it happened again I should get up and turn on the light instead of calling her to do it. If I did that and he was still there, she would know I wasn't dreaming. She told me to sleep with either of my two roommates if I wanted to. But I knew they were both homosexual, so I stayed in my own bed.

"I couldn't recall ever having met the man in person, though I've searched my memory many times. Yet I have the strangest feeling that I must have known him at one time or that I may meet him in my future—odd as that may seem to someone who has never experienced such a feeling.

"It may be important that he appeared at night. Night was the loneliest time for me as a child and teenager. I could cry and let out my feelings without anyone seeing me. I wonder if he may have been there to comfort me, not to frighten me.

"He didn't age from one time to the next—each time he seemed to be in his early twenties. He resembled me, as I look now."

I recognized that, like her father's apparition, the man in white had appeared upon her waking from sleep. The man had been there only then, and disappeared when the lights were turned on, whereas her father's apparition manifested at any time, sometimes in full daylight. The man's apparition had not spoken or moved, whereas her father's apparition spoke, and moved, and shook her bed with its legs, all of which made it seem even more like a live person.

"My first child, George, was born when I was eighteen.

"Four years later, in my second pregnancy, the baby was a breech presentation, and I had a long and difficult labor. The baby, a girl, was born at one thirty in the morning. A few hours later, before breakfast, I was lying drowsy, but awake, in a semiprivate hospital room. The baby, Heather, had been taken away to let me rest. I glanced at the blank television screen in my room and glimpsed a figure reflected there. I looked toward the place in the room where the figure reflected would have had to be standing, and I saw a boy there, aged sixteen or seventeen, standing on the windowsill inside the room. He was wearing tight, faded blue-jeans with patches on them, grubby tennis shoes that looked comfortable, a jacket, and a little silly hat of a sort a teenager might like. His hair was long and light brown. He was life-sized. The windows were very tall, so there was plenty of room for him to stand on the sill. But it made no sense. We were on the third floor, and no fire escape was outside, and I hadn't seen him cross the room, so I didn't see how he could have gotten there. I wasn't frightened and didn't call for help. I asked the woman in the next bed if she saw anyone. She said, 'Where?' I said, 'In the window.' She said, 'No.' I looked a couple more times, and he was still there. Then he was gone.

"I told the doctor about this, and he said it was the medication I was on. I had received an injection the night before to put me to sleep, and was also on pills for pain. The doctor stopped the medication.

"It was the first apparition I'd seen since I was sixteen, six years earlier. Afterward, I wondered if perhaps the face of the boy in the window was an image of what Heather would look like as a teenager, or perhaps of what Heather's future boyfriend would look like.

"During my third and last pregnancy, when I was about eighteen weeks pregnant, I began to bleed from my vagina. My obstetrician admitted me to a hospital immediately, to prevent me from miscarrying.

"One night in the hospital before I went to sleep, two men— they were probably orderlies—came to my ward and lifted a woman lying in a bed near me onto a trolley. The woman was crying pitifully and was protesting, 'I don't want to go.' The men wheeled the trolley with the woman on it through the swinging double doors at the entrance to the ward. As far as I know, the men weren't apparitions.

"I suppose the woman was being moved elsewhere—probably to the operating room—because she was about to miscarry a baby. I felt terrible thinking of her baby dying and of all the dead babies whose mothers had been wheeled through those doors.

"I went to sleep, and later awoke. The room was dark except for a light from the hall. The same two men who had taken away that other woman were standing next to my bed. I watched the men let the rails of my bed down, and as the rails were lowered, I heard them clang. I rang the nursing station to say, 'Don't let them do it.' I felt the men, one at the head of the bed and one at the foot, lift me up together with my top mattress and put me on a trolley, just as I had seen them do with the other woman. The nurse came and saw how upset I was. I begged her to tell the men not to take me away. I said the doctor had advised me to rest—to lie still, not to get up, and to call the nurse for a bedpan rather than walk to the toilet. He had said if I did all that, I'd be all right and wouldn't have to worry. And I'd done all that, I said, and I knew I was better, because the bleeding had already slowed down and I was only spotting now. While I was talking to the nurse, the men were there, though I realized later she wasn't seeing them. At some point the men were gone. [13]

"The nurse went to get my doctor. He came, and sat on my bed. I was crying. I told him what had just happened—how the men had come and tried to take me to the operating room. He said, 'It must have been the men in the hall you saw.' I said, 'No, they came to fetch me.' He asked, 'Which men?' I described them to him. One was blond, I recall now. The doctor held my hands and took his handkerchief out to wipe my tears. He said, 'Calm down. No one will hurt you or your baby.' He told me the men I described had already gone home and couldn't possibly have just come to me. He showed me in the hall the two orderlies who were now on duty. He asked, 'Are those the men?' I said, 'No.' He sat with me until I calmed down.

"Soon after that, I was discharged from the hospital. I went on with that pregnancy until nine months was up and delivered Yvonne. That was my last apparitional experience until a year later, when I first saw the apparition of my father."

As I reviewed Ruth's history, a question passed swiftly through my mind. Given her childhood history of seeing apparitions, could I—or she—be sure that she had not hallucinated her father's sexual attack upon her at ten? This is another version of a doubt I had entertained earlier about the attack. I knew there was no way to gain certainty. However, I now also knew that much else was compatible with the event having actually occurred. Besides the father's alleged sexual violation of Ruth, there were his other outbursts of violence. There was other evidence of his sexual interest in Ruth at ten. There was his sexual aggressiveness toward Jane, Ruth's younger sister, when Jane was twelve. There was his sexual interest in Mallory, the older sister, manifested by his falsely accusing her of sexual relations with boys. And, most relevantly, there was his reminding Ruth when she was twenty-one, and he was her houseguest, of his sexual assault upon her when she was ten.

I also learned that there may have been incest in the father's family of origin. "Among my father's cousins," Ruth said, "brother-sister incest has occurred with seveal couples. A father and daughter have had an ongoing sexual relationship too.

"My mother and Mallory told me that, in his early twenties, my father had sexual intercourse with his stepmother while his own father lay dying. The stepmother got pregnant and had his child. My father's real mother and father had divorced. The child, Agnes, is now a grown woman about eleven years older than me. I'd known Agnes for years before being told we were half-sisters. After hearing this story, I asked my father if it was true—he said it was."

Perhaps it is humankind's destiny to have to cope with incestuous desires. In Ruth's case, it may have been determined before she was born that the likelihood of incest actually occurring in her life was higher than it is for most people.

All the information I have so far related about Ruth's past was obtained by methods that are in no way extraordinary. I later came to be informed about more of her past by means that were, to say the least, unusual. The fresh information did not contradict anything that I have so far presented. Rather, it added to my understanding of what had already been communicated to me.

Changes

A few days after Ruth left the Crisis Centre, I went to the United States for two and a half weeks.

While I was away, a skeptical inner voice haunted me: "When Ruth tells you she's making her father appear in your office or upon your face, how do you know she's really seeing what she says she's seeing? Given her fear of seeing his apparition, she could simply be pretending to see it, without having actually made him appear."

It was possible. Only she could know what she was experiencing.

"However," a trustful voice said, "at the same time that she alleges she sees the apparition, she acts as if she sees it: she trembles, cries, blushes, perspires, wrings her hands. . . ."

"A talented actress," interrupted the skeptic, "can display fear convincingly if her role demands it. Ruth could be playing at being scared. Or, she could be thrusting herself into a fearful state without seeing a frightening image."

"Perhaps," said the trusting voice; "but you haven't known her to be capable of persuasive dramatic performances in other circumstances."

"How well do you know her?" the skeptic asked.

I did not know how good an actress she was, though I knew she had had no formal training. I knew she had been having—or said she had been having—apparitional experiences just before she had met me; allegedly, that is why she had sought my help and why she had thought she had been going crazy. I now knew she had also had—or said she had had—a history of apparitional experiences. But I had no evidence besides her testimony that her past experiences were genuine hallucinations.

I felt unable to resolve the matter just then. Later I was to come upon a means for testing whether she was hallucinating when she said she was.

Ruth had decided that while I was away she would keep a diary. One reason for keeping it was to be able to show it to me when I returned. She wanted a record of those experiences that she thought would interest me. In her first entry, she wrote that she felt "not so alone somehow," since she knew I would be reading what she would be writing. After my return to England, she could meet me only once a week, as she lived far from my office, so she continued keeping her diary.

I have added nothing to the following excerpts from her diary. In dating them, I have called the day she left the Crisis Centre "Day 1," her first full day at home "Day 2," and so on:

Day 1

Paul and I put the children to bed, and then it was time for us to sleep. Paul turned out the light and came to bed. "This should prove interesting," I said to myself.

I could see my father—his face wasn't clear—in the corner behind the door. I buried my face in the pillow. This is all I need tonight! I thought.

Paul stayed on his side of the bed and didn't try to reach

out to me. Maybe he doesn't like sharing a bed with me anymore.

I felt very insecure about falling asleep, but finally I did. The night was dark and long, and a mass of confusing dreams. I felt afraid all night.

Day 2

It's getting dark, and my nerves are shot. I'm awake and writing to keep from sleeping and dreaming.

My father laughed at me today and said, "You're back home now, no stronger or wiser than you were. You're going on twenty-six years old, but you look forty." I wonder how forty looks. He's not so pretty himself!

I'm frightened that he's still with me and still bothering me, but not as frightened as I've been.

I haven't left the house yet. I had two visitors. I don't particularly enjoy their company. I let them in anyway because I felt I should. I found I wasn't afraid.

Day 3

Last night I had many dreams. I don't recall them, but I know I kept waking up at the points when the dreams got bad. I kept going back to sleep and dreaming the same dreams again.

There was a parent-teacher meeting at the school today. I didn't attend. I didn't want to go. I was too tired to make the effort. I feel I've deserted my children, and I hate to face anyone connected with them. I made an appointment for a later day.

My father was just here. He was sitting by the radiator. Paul knew I was seeing him. I made my father disappear, and after it, I felt so tired I lay down and just went to bed.

Day 4

I think I'll write what I dreamed last night. I was all alone with my father in a room without doors or windows. Just

walls, and me, and him. I made myself scream and woke up.
Today, I'm here along with George and Yvonne. My father
is here too, sitting on the sofa. He's not talking. The cushion
he's been sitting on is crushed as if he was sitting on it. He
took a cigarette pack from his shirt pocket and popped a
cigarette from the pack. I could hear the popping, his clothes
rustling when he reached into his pocket, and his fingers
rubbing against the cigarette when he put it in his mouth.
He took out a lighter and flicked open the top. I wondered if I
would smell the lighter fluid. He was about to light the
cigarette. If he smoked it, I was going to ask George if he
smelled smoke. As if my father read my thoughts, he put the
cigarette and lighter back in his pockets, and looked at me as
if to say, "You thought I was going to light it but I didn't."

Day 5
I dreamed I was in a house built on stilts, on the beach.
There was a black cloud and a storm. I wanted to leave, but
the storm was too bad. A voice said, "It's too late for you to
get away." I was terrified.
I felt worse today than yesterday.

Day 9
My father is always moving about the house. I'll see him go
by a door, and I'll glimpse him just enough to know who it is.
He still upsets me a little, but I ignore him now.

Day 16
I've been feeling so good I haven't written in my diary.
My father woke me this morning by sitting on my bed. At
first I thought it was Paul sitting there putting on his shoes. I
hate it when my father makes me feel something real like
that. He was smiling. "Do you know why I'm here?" he
asked. "Oh, God, not you—I'm too tired," I said. I asked if
he'd been in the kitchen. He seemed disturbed by my being
so casual. "Yes," he said. "Has Paul made a pot of coffee?" I

asked. "What?" he said. I asked again. "What do you mean?" he said, and he looked confused because he wasn't used to me talking to him like that. "If the coffee is made," I said, "I'll get out of bed. If it's not, I won't." He seemed dumbfounded. He nodded his head and said, "It's made." I had to see if he was right, so I jumped out of bed and went to the kitchen. Paul had made the coffee!

I used him, as Dr. Schatzman told me to. I'll use him now every chance I get. I wish I could tell Dr. Schatzman right now, this minute. I feel so happy. I haven't felt so great in a long time.

Day 17

I saw my father while I was in the bathtub. I was frightened, which he enjoyed. I felt terrible about his looking at me, but I didn't try to cover my body. Then I decided not to let him enjoy it. I asked him to get me a towel. I didn't really believe he would. "Hurry up, I'm cold," I said, as hateful as I could. "What's the matter?" he said. "Are you ashamed of the stretch marks on your tummy?" "Hell, no!" I said and laughed. "I'm proud of the kids who put them there!" "I don't care who put them there," he said, "they look awful." "Well, I like them," I said. "Nobody asked you in here to look at them. It's my house, my bathroom, my tummy, and my stretch marks. Get out of here and out of my life!" I threw the soap at him. "You little bitch!" he said. He opened the door to walk out, and I felt a draft of air. I walked over to the towel rack, and got a towel. All this time I was standing up to him and not showing him my fear and disgust. When he was gone, it all hit me at once. I felt sick, and I had to kneel by the toilet to throw up.

I really don't like my stretch marks, and I think he knew it.

Why did Dr. Schatzman have to leave me? I'm angry he's away. I need him so badly.

Day 22

My father has been going into Yvonne's room. I haven't been going in there to see if he's harming her. The reason why is I think he wants for me to believe he's real and for me to check on Yvonne. But I know he's not, so I haven't been. Last night I had one of the best dreams I've ever had. It was a turning point for me. The dream had a terrible beginning. I dreamed my father was screaming at me. He had his fist clenched and he was fixing to be violent. I was frightened and called for Dr. Schatzman. My father said Dr. Schatzman won't come, that he was away in body and mind. He started removing his trousers. Dr. Schatzman came in, and asked why I was crying and trembling. What got said after that is this:

MY FATHER (*to Dr. Schatzman*): What are you doing here?

DR. SCHATZMAN: I was invited, which is more than I can say for you.

MY FATHER (*laughs, and says to me*): Your psychiatrist is as crazy as you are, because he is seeing me and talking to me now. (*Laughs for a long time*).

ME: Do you really see him?

DR. SCHATZMAN: Yes. You've made an image for both of us to see and to deal with as we want.

MY FATHER: If you're so goddamned great, Doc, let's see you get rid of me. I'm not leaving.

DR. SCHATZMAN: You'll leave when Ruth and I decide. But we're not through with you yet.

MY FATHER: What gave you the idea I'd let you do anything? (*He pointed to me.*) She's crazy. You can't believe that little fucker. (*He looked at Dr. Schatzman.*) And you're crazy too. (*He laughed.*) Well, get started, Great Doctor. Move mountains, divide the sea. (*He laughed.*)

DR. SCHATZMAN: You're only here because Ruth allows you

here. You can't harm her or me because you don't
exist. She has created you with her unconscious
mind. You're only a product of her creative thinking
or imagination. She's using your body or form to
relieve feelings of her own that she doesn't even know
about. Putting it one way, you're just an outlet.

ME: No, Dr. Schatzman, that's not true. I don't think or feel
the terrible things he says about you. Please don't
believe that. Those feelings couldn't be mine.

DR. SCHATZMAN: Are you sure? Maybe the feelings he shows
are feelings of yours that you don't think are allowed.

I awoke. I went to the bathroom and ran the tub full of hot
water. Then I just lay in the tub for a long time, and cried,
and laughed, and cried.

Something happened last night. But what? How could I
have allowed such a gross figure to have entered my life? I
wonder if he's there because he's a very important part of me.
Not a good part, but still an important part.

A few days later I returned to England and saw her.

She and Paul had made love twice, she told me. "It wasn't as
sweet as it has sometimes been, but we both reached a climax
each time." She was delighted about having asked her father's
apparition if the coffee was made and about the dream just
reported. The remarks in her dream about the relation between
the apparition and her "unconscious mind" fascinated me. They
resembled my actual views. I probably had implied to her that I
thought the apparition's hostility to me might really be her own
unconscious hostility, but I had never straightforwardly told her
so. Perhaps she had heard such an idea from someone at the
Crisis Centre. Perhaps it was a product of her creative thinking,
and in her dream she was having me express her own unconscious
understanding.

To her relief, the apparition did not manifest after this dream
for nineteen days in her dreams or waking life. This was its

longest absence since her first experience of it. She was feeling
"over the worst," she said, and no longer frightened.
Then, as she wrote in her diary:

Day 41

It happened again. I'd just gone to bed and was lying
awake. I hadn't fallen asleep yet. Paul was asleep. His hair
was grayish looking, not its usual brown color. I felt like
running from him. My hands started to tremble. I pulled the
sheet away from his face. He was lying there laughing. It was
my father, not Paul. I reached out and shook him to see who
would awaken and talk to me: Paul or my father. He awoke,
and started looking like Paul. I feel so desperate. I had
thought it was over.

Though she had been premature in having supposed "it was
over," her desperate feelings seemed to me unwarranted. Her
sexual relations with Paul were infrequent and not as "sweet" as
she wished. However, most of the evidence of depression and
anxiety she had reported when she had first come to me was gone.
She was generally feeling calmer than she had in a long while.

She had achieved a remarkable degree of symptom relief in a
brief time, although neither she nor I understood why the
apparition had begun to harass her in the first place.

Twenty-five days after the date of the last diary entry I have
quoted, Ruth was sitting in my office looking relaxed and
cheerful.

"As I got to the door of your office today," she said, "a couple
was leaving. I recognized them because we used to live in the
same neighborhood, although we'd never spoken to each other.
The woman poked the man in the ribs and I heard her say, 'She
sees Dr. Schatzman in psychotherapy too.' I said to them loudly,
'I do, but I'm not crazy.'"

I chuckled. "But she wasn't saying you are."

"I know." She settled back in her seat. "I haven't been

experiencing the apparition. I've been trying to keep it from appearing. I want my experience of it to be over."

She seemed to become tense. "I've been dreading that you might make my father appear here today. I don't want to see him."

It was odd that she thought I could make her father appear. I could only ask her to do it, and if she didn't want to, I couldn't make her. I didn't comment about her choice of words, though I decided I might at another time.

"I've been reviewing some literature on apparitions and hallucinations," I said. "From what I've found, it seems that the ability to produce a lifelike apparition at will is rare. How do you feel about that?"

"It must mean I'm some kind of nut."

"But you told that couple you weren't crazy. Was it yourself you were trying to convince? I think you just have an unusual capacity for imaginative creation."

What I next said had crucial consequences for all that subsequently occurred. "Why don't you produce an apparition of someone else, someone you've had a friendlier relationship with than you've had with your father? Perhaps such an apparition could be your ally."

She was silent for a few seconds. "I don't know if I could."

"You'll only find out if you try."

Again she was silent.

"What about creating an apparition of your mother?"

"I think not." She said it quickly, curtly, as if to say, "And I don't want you to pursue the matter by asking, 'Why?'" She continued: "My best friend, who's been more like a sister, is Becky. We've been close for nearly our whole lives. I haven't seen her in over two years." She hesitated.

"Why don't you try to see an apparition of her?"

She was sitting facing me. She turned toward an empty chair and stared at it for a few seconds. "No, I can't there. I want to look at the doorway."

The door, on her left, was open and gave access to a hallway. She turned to face the doorway and stared at it for about twenty seconds. "I can see Becky's form, but not her face or flesh. Her face seems to be behind a haze. She's staying in the doorway, not entering the room. I can't tell what she's wearing. I can see her legs. Her hair is longer than it used to be. She's laughing, perhaps because I'm talking about her hair. Seeing her feels good."

Ruth paused. "She's gone. She faded faster than she came. My concentration broke, and she faded. If I'd tried harder, I could have kept her here longer."

Ruth sighed. "Seeing her has made me feel happier than I've felt in days. It's almost as if I'd had a visit from her. She seemed pleased to be here. I'm shaking inside, like I do when I see my father, but it's not with fear. Maybe I'm shaking because I'm excited. I feel cold too."

"Did you smell anything?"

"No, but I didn't think to."

"How would you feel about trying it again?"

"All right." She stared at the doorway. "I can't do it as easily this time."

Fifteen seconds passed. "Do you know who's coming into the picture?" she said.

"No."

She continued to peer at the doorway. "My father. He's plainer than Becky was, but not as plain as he's been. I see his clothes and hair. I can make him fade, and I can bring him back with no trouble. But I can't make her appear."

She turned to me. "Let's not do it anymore. I don't feel well."

She was silent for a few seconds. She seemed to be relaxing. "Nothing about that doorway changed between Becky's appearance and my father's, but when he appeared, the whole atmosphere was different somehow. It became unpleasant. I can't separate my feelings toward an apparition of him from my feelings toward him. I'm afraid of him in real life and I'm afraid of his apparition."

I was pleased that Ruth had enjoyed Becky's appearance. Ideas crowded into my mind for helping Ruth by using her capacity to produce apparitions.

Meanwhile another dialogue was going on inside me. As before, it began with the skeptical voice. "May I remind you that you don't know whether she's really seeing what she says she's seeing. I'm not suggesting she's lying. Rather, for the sake of pleasing you, she could be supposing she's having an experience that she isn't really having."

"How could that be?" I wondered.

"She might be experiencing Becky in imagination, as you or I might imagine someone, but believing that Becky is appearing to her as a real person.

"Yes, Ruth might be," I thought. "But if so, she's doing something very similar indeed to what she says she's doing: seeing Becky and knowing that what she's seeing is a hallucination." Certainly Ruth was eager to please me. But that did not in itself give grounds for skepticism about her testimony.

Once again I recognized that I could not be sure whether Ruth's accounts of her experiences were accurate. But the same applied, I reasoned, to anyone's description of any hallucinatory experience.

My next session with Ruth was two weeks later. She was wearing lipstick and a bit of mascara for the first time since I'd known her. She had pulled some of her hair back and tied a thin red band round it. She seemed to have lost some weight too.

"I have two things to tell you," she began. "The first one is this. Paul was away a few days on business. One of the nights he was away I went to bed. As I walked into the bedroom, I saw someone's form in our bed. That's not unusual; the children sometimes sleep with me when Paul is away. None of the children had mentioned they'd be sleeping there, but they don't always tell me.

"I turned the light on, and there, sitting on the bed, was an apparition of my father! His chest was bare, and he had the sheet pulled up to his waist. I had the terrifying feeling that he was naked. A soft scream came out of my mouth before I could stifle it. My body was trembling. 'What are you doing?' I asked. 'Waiting for you to come to bed,' he said. He patted the bed next to where he was lying.

"I ran into my daughter Heather's room and got into bed with her. I didn't feel we were in danger. I mean, I knew this was an apparition. But I just couldn't bring myself to sleep in my own bed that night.

"The next morning I looked into my room, and he was gone. The bed was still made from the day before. It hadn't been disturbed."

I decided to try a fresh approach. "About two months ago, you dreamed that I told your father's apparition that it was expressing your own unconscious feelings. Let's suppose that view were correct. Then the experience you've just described might be expressing your sexual desire toward your father, or perhaps your memory of having felt that way in the past. According to that reasoning, you really are or have been sexually interested in him, but instead of letting yourself feel that interest, you create an apparition of him, who displays sexual interest in you. You displace your feelings onto the apparition."

"Do you really believe that?" Her voice was mocking, and her eyes seemed to say that if, after all this time, I could entertain the notion that she found her father sexually attractive, I must be naive or insensitive.

My reply moved sideways, neither retreating nor advancing. "I don't know whether I believe it or not. It's plausible. Whether it's true is another matter."

"I don't find my father sexually attractive. Ever since the rape I've found him revolting and disgusting." Her tone seemed to say, "And that's final."

"And before the rape?"

"I may have found him attractive at times. But not sexually. At that age I wasn't aware of sexual feelings toward anyone."

I thought that if she had repressed her sexual feelings toward her father, she would reject my interpretation, even if it were correct. On the other hand, my interpretation might be wrong, and her reason for rejecting it right.

"What was the second thing you wanted to tell me?" I asked.

"I've managed to see Becky completely. At first my father kept interfering, by appearing in the place where I was trying to make her appear. But then I succeeded. I could see her clothes. They were in a different style than the clothes she used to wear. Again, her hair was long. Otherwise she looked like she had when I last saw her. She hadn't aged. I said, 'Hello.' She replied, 'Hello.' That was all we said.

"When I next produced her, I was having a bubble bath. The bathtub is the only place where I'm alone with my thoughts. She was wearing blue jeans, a pink sweater, and an unbuttoned vest that matched her jeans. Her fingernails were polished, exactly the same shade as her sweater. A fingernail on her left hand was broken. Her lipstick was light pink. She was perfectly groomed.

"She laughed and said, 'Who do you think you are, inviting all these people in to see you while you're in a bubble bath—some movie queen?'

"I said, 'But you're my only guest.'

"'That's true,' she replied. We laughed together."

I interrupted Ruth. "What did you think she meant by 'all those people in to see you?'"

"I don't know. Maybe she was referring to the previous visit of my father's apparition.

"Then Becky pulled down the toilet lid to sit on. The two of us used to talk like that when we were kids, me lying in the bath and her sitting on the toilet lid.

"She told me she was glad to see me. She asked if I remembered certain things we'd done together as children. I did. I said I'd been missing her and all the fun we used to have. I wasn't speaking out loud, because I expected that, as I'd created her, she'd know my thoughts.

"She said, 'We'll make up for the time we haven't seen each other.'

"I said, 'I've been writing about my life, which you used to encourage me to do.'

"'You've gained some weight since I last saw you.'

"'Yes,' I admitted.

"She asked, 'Have you been exercising to lose weight?'

"I replied, 'I've been doing sit-ups and leg-raising exercises.'

"She said, 'I'm happy and feeling close to God.' She looked happy.

"Then she said she was leaving, and she walked out. As she did, the door opened and a cold draft of air came from the doorway, as if the door had actually opened. The draft made me sink deeper in the tub to get warm. Then the door closed. When she had gone, I noticed the toilet lid was back in its original place.

"I felt tired and had a headache from the effort of producing her. I also felt excited, glad, and uplifted. I knew Becky hadn't really been there, but I felt as I would have if she really had."

I didn't try to restrain my pleasure at her accomplishment. "That's excellent. I'm delighted."

I was impressed with how her skill as an observer of her own experience had sharpened. Perhaps what had sharpened was her skill at knowing what sorts of observations would impress me, but the result was the same.

"I'm delighted too," she said. "There's another thing. I tried to make an apparition of you, and I succeeded a bit. I'm going to practice."

I nodded and lifted my eyebrows approvingly. "I'm looking forward to hearing what happens."

"I realize now I've had this ability all my life. I've even somehow known all along it was there. But I'd never used it. Maybe I was afraid people would think I was crazy or a witch. If I were living four hundred years ago, I'd have been burned, wouldn't I?"

"If you'd been indiscreet and attracted the wrong people's attention, perhaps."

"The person I worry about is Paul. He's concerned about my making apparitions. I couldn't go on if he disapproved."

"Does he disapprove?"

"It's all very strange to him."

I wondered if she was thinking it all very strange herself and attributing that thinking to him; or if both of them felt that way. Possibly she felt Paul and I were in conflict with each other—he opposing her experiments and I encouraging them; if so, it might be because she was in conflict herself about them.

"Is Paul here today?" I asked.

"He's in the waiting room."

"Would you like to ask him to come in?"

"All right." She left the room.

She entered with Paul behind her. As usual, he was dressed casually and groomed neatly. He and I nodded, said "Hi!" and smiled to each other. I have sometimes learned much about a person's state of mind by watching how he or she enters a room and sits down. But watching Paul, I could tell nothing.

"Shall we exchange views on where things stand?" I said to him. "How are you finding Ruth?"

He smiled. "Much better. Relaxed, doing things, going out. She's her old self, almost."

"I find she's better too." I thought it best to agree out loud about something that pleased us both before going on to the next matter. "Ruth told me you're having doubts about her recent activities with apparitions."

"I'd never heard of anyone deliberately producing them before."

He seemed to be measuring every word, making it hard for me to gauge the quality of his underlying feeling. Again I chose to express agreement. "Neither have I."

"Could her fooling around be dangerous?" His calling it "fooling around" seemed patronizing, though it might have been an expression of worry. "Could it bring on another emotional crisis?" he asked.

"I don't wish to see her in another emotional crisis any more than you do. I can't guarantee she'll continue to do well, but there's no reason to believe she won't. As to what you call her 'fooling around,' I've never had experience with someone just like her before. However, I think it's safe and even therapeutic for her to bring under her own power an experience that used to frighten her. Exposing people to things they fear or have feared is generally harmless. And the more one gets used to facing something that one has been afraid of, the stronger one becomes. Moreover Ruth's attitude toward the apparitions has changed. Earlier she had believed she was going crazy; she was scared, withdrawn, and unhappy. Now she can see the apparitions as expressions of a creative talent. They're no longer intruders. She's even feeling playful toward them. Yogis produce unusual experiences all the time and set store by them, and they don't usually go mad or develop psychiatric symptoms."

Though I was talking about "she" and "her" as if Ruth were not there, I occasionally looked at her. I was speaking to Paul about her, but guessed I was addressing a part of her that had been having doubts.

No one said anything for a few seconds. "Sounds reasonable," Paul said.

"I suggest," I added, "that if Ruth notices an alarming change in her state of mind, or if you or I see a worrying shift in her behavior, we notify each other."

They both nodded.

One reason for her continuing to create apparitions was to explore the characteristics of apparitional phenomena, and I now thought it timely to review what she had reported about them and to pose some questions.

Ruth had distinguished two sorts of experiences. Sometimes she formed an image of her father appearing in her mother's living room, in a car, or in some other surroundings where she remembered having seen him before. In these experiences, in which her eyes were open or closed, she saw him in her "mind's eye" or with her memory. She was imagining him in the same sense that most people mean when they speak of imagining something. Other times, with her eyes open, she saw her father amidst the persons and objects of her actual environment, "as I'd see you or as I'd see anyone who was there with me." These were hallucinations—"seeing things that aren't there," as she said.[14] She could easily discriminate between the two kinds of experience.

Her problem, at first, had been to tell the difference between persons she was apparently seeing who were not really there and persons she was actually seeing who were really there. The reason for the problem was the astonishing resemblance of the apparitions to living people.[15]

The persons she hallucinated looked as real to her as live persons, and were as clear and vivid in all details. Her father's apparition had gray hairs in his eyebrows, and she could discern individual teeth in his mouth. Becky's apparition had worn nail polish on her fingernails, and one of her fingernails had been broken. So exactly could an apparition imitate a normal figure that the first time she had seen her father's apparition she had initially thought it was her father.

"I don't go to the apparitions, they come to me," Ruth once said. They would manifest in whatever place she happened to be. Never had she seen an apparition in a special area of its own, such as in a space seemingly cut out of a wall or on the polished surface of a wardrobe.

The figures she hallucinated would "bring only themselves," she said. They were never accompanied by a hallucinated environment. In this respect her hallucinatory experiences differed from those of a dream, in which an entire scene is invented.

The apparitions would walk on the floor, not walk in the air or fly. They related normally to the features of her surroundings: they walked around furniture rather than through it, and sat on chairs, couches, beds, or toilet lids. When she looked away from an apparition, she stopped seeing it. If she left a room in which her father's apparition was present, on her return she might or might not find the apparition still there. If she stayed in the room with it, it would eventually leave, usually by walking through a doorway, not by walking through a wall or by simply vanishing. And in leaving, it would generally open a door that was closed, and then close it again.

Occasionally an apparition had given itself away, by acting as an apparition is traditonally supposed to act, rather than as a person does. For instance, the father's apparition had once left a room by passing right through a closed door. Another time it had placed itself in a room with her, and when she had gone to a different room, it had arrived there before she did, without having passed her along the way. However, this sort of behavior, which made obvious the apparition's nonmaterial nature, was most uncommon in Ruth's experience.

When her father's apparition had manifested in other people's presence, it had taken their presence into account and had related to them as a person might. If someone was talking with Ruth, the apparition would follow the conversation by turning its head and nodding, and sometimes by making relevant remarks.

The apparitions had worn clothes and had dressed suitably. When the father's apparition had manifested in Ruth's bed once late in the evening, it had been bare-chested, which might be expected of someone lying in bed at that hour. The apparition of the father, who in real life smoked cigarettes, had once taken from his pocket cigarettes and a lighter which had looked real to Ruth.

The apparition of the adolescent boy standing on the windowsill, who had manifested after Ruth's delivery of Heather, had been reflected on a blank television screen as a real person would have been.

It is said that seeing is believing. Ruth's other senses had conspired together with her eyes to make disbelief in the evidence of her eyes difficult. She had heard the apparitions make sounds that real people make, and the sounds had been clear. She had heard familiar voices when the apparitions of her father and Becky had spoken. When her father's apparition had talked at the same time as a person had been talking, she had found it hard to hear the person. When she had seen her father's apparition take out a cigarette to light, she had heard accompanying popping and rustling noises. She had heard footsteps and the rubbing of trouser legs behind her when she thought her father had been following her.

When an apparition had seemed to open the bathroom door, she had felt a draft of cold air. Once, she had felt her bed shake before she had seen the legs of her father's apparition knocking against it. Another time, she had been awakened by feeling someone sitting down upon her bed, and then had seen it was her father's apparition. While pregnant with her third child, she had hallucinated in the hospital not only the sight and sound but also the bodily feeling of two orderlies lifting her off the bed.

She had smelled the odor of her father's apparition a few times, and it had persisted once, even after the apparition had left the room.

How then could she distinguish an apparition from a living person? Suppose she were among a group of people. How was she to know if one of them might be an apparition and not real? An apparition could be mixed in with the real people and not be noticed.

She posed the same question herself in a dream: "Pop music was playing. You, your wife, Laura, Andrea, my father, my grandmother, and some other people I didn't know were holding hands and dancing around my bed. At this moment I knew I was asleep and dreaming, because I knew the head of my bed was against the wall and no one could be dancing around it. Yet I continued the dream because I wanted to see how it was going to turn out."

The head of her bed was, in fact, against the wall.

"Next I dreamed that I sat up in bed and asked all of you, 'What are you doing?' You said, 'Ruth, all of us are real except for one of us. We want you to tell us which one of us is an apparition.' I said, 'That's crazy. This is a dream. None of you are real. I'm the only one here.' You laughed and said, 'But are you sure?' One lady spoke up, 'Would you like to dance?' I said, 'Yes.' She said, 'Come and join the circle here.' She let go someone's hand so I could enter the circle. When I got to the circle, I saw I'd have to hold my father's hand. I said, 'I don't think I want to dance.' You said, 'It's all right, Ruth, just make him disappear.' I took your hand and laughed. I turned to my father and said, 'Do you ever get the feeling you're not wanted?' I told him to leave, which he did.

"I guess he was the apparition you were talking about."

If Ruth were in this situation in waking life, difficulties could present themselves. Suppose, for instance, the same scenario as the one in the dream were to happen, but the figure of her father were to tell her to make me disappear. And suppose she tried to, and succeeded! This might not, after all, be beyond her powers, as she had obscured from her view real walls and real objects when the figures of the apparitions had moved in front of them. How would she then know if I were real? How would she know who was real? Might she have seen an apparition among a group of live people without suspecting it of being an apparition?

It was impossible to know how many apparitions, if any, had passed through her experience without her suspecting their true nature.

Only upon her seeing a figure that she suspected was apparitional did the problem arise of distinguishing the apparitional from the real. Upon seeing a youth's figure standing in the window of her hospital room, she had doubted that a real person could be standing in such an unlikely place. Upon seeing her father's figure sitting at her dining-room table, she had doubted that he could have afforded the cost of a trip to England. These doubts had led her to conceive that the figures might be apparitional. She had surmised more than once that a given figure was apparitional because of its manifesting inside a locked house; a live person could not have entered without a key, or without ringing a doorbell or knocking on a door, which this figure had not done. Apparitions that manifested outdoors or in an unlocked place might escape her suspicions if other clues to their real character were absent. One reason the apparitions of the two hospital orderlies had fooled her so thoroughly was that they had manifested in a hospital ward, a place where the orderlies ordinarily appeared.

The defining quality of the apparitions she had so far experienced was that they had gone unnoticed by everyone else. This is what had consistently marked them off from live persons. She had come to realize that certain figures were apparitional only upon discovering that other people had not experienced them. She had learned to rely on this quality of the apparitions as distinctive; once she had come to conjecture that a given figure was an apparition she would ascertain that it was an apparition by turning to another person. So far, no one had corroborated what she saw—which did not mean no one ever would. Perhaps if an apparition manifested in the company of a sufficiently sensitive person, that person might see or hear it, even though other persons would not. Admittedly this seemed unlikely—but could I be sure it was impossible?

Recently she had become aware of another feature of the apparitions that distinguished them from live persons. They left behind them no trace of having been present. This was consistent with their being products of her own mind. Though they had sometimes seemed to make material changes in their environments during the period of their manifestations, these changes had vanished upon their departure. She could use this property of her hallucinatory experiences as a means of identifying a given figure as apparitional, but only after the figure's disappearance. Could an apparition leave behind it a physical mark that she would continue to notice after its departure? Might someone else be able to notice that mark? It seemed unlikely. However, all she or I could say with certainty is that this had not occurred, as far as she now knew.

I have pointed out that the apparitions characteristically blocked from Ruth's view whatever objects were behind them. When an apparition moved around a room, the area hidden from her view moved with the apparition, just as if the apparition were a live person. This quality of the apparitions intrigued me. It meant that her apparitional experiences were being precisely and skillfully coordinated with the inhibition of her normal visual experiences.

Once, while taking a bath at home, she asked an apparition of Becky to put some toothpaste on her toothbrush, since she wanted to brush her teeth after her bath. The toothbrush and toothpaste were, in fact, really there. She watched Becky pick up the toothpaste tube, remove the cap, and squeeze some toothpaste onto the toothbrush; Becky squeezed the middle of the tube. The tube had been full, and Ruth wished Becky had squeezed it from the bottom; but the tube was now already compressed. Ruth observed—and here is the point which excited my curiosity—that from the moment she hallucinated Becky's hands picking up the toothbrush and the tube, the real toothbrush and tube disappeared from view. Ruth was sure of this, because she looked at the particular place where she had previously seen them—and they were not there. Here again the inhibition of a normal visual experience dovetailed with a hallucinatory experience.

When the apparition had left, Ruth climbed out of the tub to brush her teeth. She turned toward where she had seen the apparition lay down the toothbrush and tube for her, but they were not there. She saw that the toothbrush and toothpaste were back in their original position, the toothbrush with no toothpaste on it, and the toothpaste tube uncompressed. In observance of apparitional customs, the apparition had left behind it no material evidence of having been present.

In all the experiences which Ruth had come to recognize as hallucinatory, whether she had hallucinated objects—or, as in the experience just related, the movement of objects—the objects had been directly associated with the hallucinatory figure of a person, for example, the clothes worn by the apparitions, the cigarette and lighter handled by her father's apparition, and the toothbrush and toothpaste in the experience with Becky's apparition. Ruth had no reason to believe she had ever hallucinated objects on their own (that is to say unassociated with an apparition), or intangible objects such as light or mist. This does not necessarily mean she had not hallucinated any of these; only that if she had, she had not discovered her experiences of them to be hallucinatory.

In each experience that she had identified as hallucinatory, she had hallucinated a person. Except for the two hospital orderlies, she had always hallucinated one person at a time.

Her hallucinations had varied in duration from a second or two to about fifteen or twenty minutes at the longest.

The apparitions' behavior had generally accorded with the usual behavior of the individuals they were representing. The father's apparition had bullied, mocked, and abused her. Becky's apparition had been friendly and pleasant. The apparitions of the hospital orderlies, who had tried to move Ruth, had done what orderlies normally do. The feelings the various apparitions had called forth in her had usually resembled the feelings she would have had, had the live persons rather than their apparitions been present.

One other attribute of the apparitions is noteworthy: both the father and Becky in their apparitional forms seemed not to have aged since Ruth had seen them in the flesh two or three years earlier—though Becky's hair was longer. This suggests that perhaps the apparitions were a product of Ruth's memory of the people concerned.

Many questions about the apparitions remained. Would an apparition allow itself to be reflected in a mirror? To be photographed? To have its voice tape-recorded? To be seen or heard by someone other than Ruth? Perhaps the apparitions might be disposed to manifest only to someone who was, like Ruth, inclined to perceive them; or to a child. If an apparition permitted Ruth to touch it, would it feel solid or like empty space? Would it cast a shadow? Would an apparition of someone other than Ruth's father or Becky manifest if Ruth bade it to? Might an apparition communicate information to her about the world, about other people, or about herself that she could not obtain otherwise? I felt sure that as the apparitions disclosed more of their properties to us, we would think of more questions.

As a child I sometimes felt while walking alone in the woods that I was in a place where no human being had ever been before. I imagined that if I stepped far enough into the untrodden upon, I might meet up with something strange and extraordinary. And then the sight of an old campfire site or some graffiti engraved on tree bark would end my reverie. I wondered now if anyone besides Ruth and me had ever traversed the same ground we were now treading upon?

I considered the possibility that she might lose her powers. They might leave as mysteriously and as quickly as they had arrived. Or, her interest might wane. Meanwhile, however, her enthusiasm and curiosity were equal to mine.

She and I agreed to talk by telephone every morning at seven. That way she could tell me any dreams she recalled from the night before, while they were fresh. And she could also narrate to me any new experiences with her "gang"—her nickname for the apparitions. On one of those phone calls she introduced herself as "your roving, not raving, reporter."

She now started to spend more time experimenting with the apparitions. She wrote in her diary:

Apparitions used to be a dreadful and abnormal part of my daily life. I hadn't dared to talk about them. Now I've learned that although they're unusual, they don't mean I'm mentally ill. I don't know what they do mean though.

Working and playing with them can be tiring. If I do it for a long time, it becomes harder and harder to do. Sometimes it drains me so much that I have to lie down and rest, usually with a headache. But I feel an excitement too, which hangs around afterward. My body feels different when I make an apparition, though I can't describe exactly how. I do know that during it I find it hard to prevent my body from shaking. If I manage to control my hands, I lose control over my stomach or knees. Perhaps it's because I'm not a very brave sort of person to start with.

With Dr. Schatzman's help, I trust I can learn from these experiences. I hope new doors will be opened, and perhaps torn completely away.

She got Paul to join in her experiments. Once, she produced an apparition of her father, and tried to have it hold Paul's hand to see if Paul could feel anything. She saw it grasp Paul's hand, but Paul felt nothing.

Another time she solicited a visit from the apparition dressed in white that had called upon her five times in her childhood. Before she did, she had to "get up the courage," she said. "Maybe with the knowledge that I now have, I won't be as frightened of him as I had been as a child." As was becoming her habit, she attempted it while taking a bath. She asked Paul to be in the bathroom with her, in case she needed him. Her cocker spaniel, Linda, was in the room too. Her diary read:

> I was just beginning to see that man I had seen as a child, when Linda started having a fit. She was running all over the bathroom and barked so bad, I had to stop. She stayed upset for a good five minutes after it was over.
> I shook something terrible. I was tearful, although I didn't actually cry. I was nervous the rest of the night.

Two nights later Ruth had a dream, which she told me on one of our early-morning telephone conversations:

> In the dream I say to you that the man dressed in white who I'd seen as a child still worries me. You want to know why he does. I tell you that he's somehow connected with my life, but I'm worried because I don't know who he is. In that case, you say, I should find out who he is. I say I don't know how to do that. You suggest I make him appear, and then ask him who he is. I say I'd like you to come with me and ask him for me. You say that since I'm the one who needs the information, I should ask myself. I agree, and, while I'm still dreaming, I decide I'll try when I wake up.

When she did awaken she found she "didn't have the courage" to bring forth the apparition. As events were to turn out, she never succeeded in obtaining a visit from it, though from time to time she thought she wanted one.

Eventually she was to use a most unusual means in gaining a fresh perspective on who that apparition represented.

*   *   *

One afternoon I was explaining something to her in my office. She interrupted: "Someone else is in the room with us." If she had a talent that was lacking in others, she was now having a chance to flaunt it. At that moment I was not her psychiatrist, but simply a friend with underdeveloped powers of visualization.

"Your father," I said.

"No. Guess again."

"Becky."

She blushed a bit. She seemed embarrassed at enjoying the inviolability of her experience. "No. It's you."

"Where?" With my head and eyes I indicated a chair near her, to her left. "There?"

"No. Over in that chair, in the corner."

There was a chair just to my left. I turned and looked. I saw no one. "What is he—or should I say 'I'?—wearing?"

"He's dressed like you." In order to check, she scanned me and then the figure to my left all over. "Just like you. The same jacket, shirt, trousers, socks, and shoes."

I looked to my left again. "How is he sitting?" I was slightly slouched in my chair, my hands folded over my lower abdomen, my legs outstretched and crossed at the ankles.

"Not the same as you. He's sitting up more in his chair, and he has one leg crossed over the other as you sometimes do. Also, his hands are separated."

"Is what is on my right side on his right side or on his left? Does he resemble me or a mirror image of me? I'm wearing a wristwatch on my left hand, and the tooth of my belt buckle goes from my left to my right. What about him?"

She looked back and forth from the chair to me a few times.

"He's the same as you."

"What would happen if I got up and went over to sit in his chair?"

"I don't know."

"I'll do it and find out."

I slowly got up from my chair and started to walk across the carpet to my left.

She stared at the chair on my left. "He's sitting there, not moving." Still staring, she gasped softly. Then she giggled and put her hand over her mouth as if to suppress a more robust laugh.

"What's happening? Why are you laughing?" I asked.

"For a second, I thought you were going to sit on him, but just when you reached his chair, he got up. He's walking over to your chair now."

"Where is he?"

"Passing in front of you. When he's in front of you, I can't see the part of you that's behind him."

I sat down in the chair on the left.

"He's sitting down now in your chair." She gestured with her eyes toward the chair I had been sitting in before.

The apparition and I had changed places.

"Let's see what happens," I said, "if I get up and return to my original chair. This time I'll walk nearer to you, so if he gets up and walks back toward his chair, he'll be behind me. We'll see if I block out your seeing him."

I got up, and walked toward Ruth before veering right.

At virtually the same time that she saw me rise from my chair, she saw the apparition rise from its chair. As I moved to my right, it moved to its left, back toward its original chair. When I passed in front of it, I blocked her seeing it. As I sat down in my chair, it sat down in its chair. Again we had switched chairs.

The apparition, like the apparition of Ruth's father and of Becky, had taken account of the ongoing situation around it. In not allowing itself to be sat upon, and in taking my seat when I took its seat, it had displayed intelligent behavior.

Would the apparition be reflected in a mirror? I fetched a full-length mirror from the next room. I set the mirror against the wall facing Ruth. I asked her to direct the apparition to stand up and to walk to the mirror.

"It's doing it. It's in front of the mirror now, facing it. I can see its reflection clearly."

I stood up and walked toward the mirror too, so that both I and the apparition would be reflected at the same time; she could then compare the two reflected images. I drew near the mirror.

"Oh!" she said, as if warning me, but also in amusement. "When you and he come near enough to touch, I expect you to bump each other. You just almost did."

I was now standing facing the mirror; presumably, the apparition was standing next to me, also facing the mirror. I put my arm around what I supposed might be the apparition's shoulder."

She smiled. "The two reflections are equally clear. Both reflections are wearing their wristwatches on the same side, and their belt buckles are going the same way too."

"Does the apparition's reflection in the mirror block out the reflection of objects in the room behind it?"

"Yes."

This meant that the apparition was inhibiting her seeing one set of objects, and its reflection was inhibiting her seeing the reflection of another set, just as a real person's reflection would.

I was feeling delighted with our progress. I grabbed what I thought might be the apparition's hand, announced that I was going to dance with the apparition, and did a fox-trot around the room with an imaginary partner. Ruth said the apparition was dancing with me!

She and I arranged to meet again in four days' time, on a Thursday evening. She would come into London and stay in a hotel near my office so that we could spend a long weekend working together. Paul would look after the children.

Another idea occurred to me. Now that she had brought forth apparitions of her father, Becky, and me, I wondered if she could also produce one of herself. I said this to her in one of our early-morning telephone talks. She said she would attempt it later that day.

I thought that an apparition of Ruth might be able to tell us things about Ruth that would add to our knowledge of her, though I did not mention this.

Her diary for that day, which she showed me on the weekend, read:

It took about two hours of continuous trying to produce an apparition of myself. It was so hard. At first I couldn't see her but for a moment or two at a time. Finally I did learn to do it.

I decided to experiment and play some games. I had the apparition sit across the room from me. I felt I was looking at someone who knew more about me than I knew about myself. I watched it closely. I tried to see if it was breathing, but I couldn't tell. The eyes fascinated me. Could I be looking through them into myself? A calm seemed to flow between us, from one to the other.

It was very tiring, and before long I had to take a nap.

While I was sleeping, I had a dream. Paul was in the dream insisting that I do an apparition of myself. I didn't want to. I wanted to rest and sleep. At this point I knew I was dreaming.

Dr. Schatzman spoke (I hadn't realized he was there until this point). He said, "Don't you want to get to know this apparition of yourself?" I started to cry and said, "No. I'm too tired." Dr. Schatzman said, "Are you afraid this apparition is angry?" I was crying so hard that it took a lot of effort to speak. I knew I was afraid and I knew why. I said, "Dr. Schatzman, I know she is angry, very angry, and I don't dare let that anger out of her. I'm afraid she'll behave like my daddy did. The anger is like a great big ball of fire. If it starts to roll, I don't think I could stop it. I'm really talking about myself, you know." Dr. Schatzman said, "I know." Tears were getting into my mouth. They were salty tasting.

Paul cupped his hand over the side of my face and said, "I love you." I asked, "Could you love me when I'm full of hate and anger?" Dr. Schatzman said, "He already does. Besides, you mustn't keep your feelings from being released. Feel the anger. Don't suppress it any longer. You're not your daddy.

It's one thing to be angry and another to be crazy." I said, "I know Paul better than you do. He won't love someone like that, Dr. Schatzman." My legs wouldn't hold me up any longer, and I fell to my knees. I laid my head upon Dr. Schatzman's lap, and pounded my fist on his chair. I felt in danger of losing everything I had. I couldn't make anyone understand. Dr. Schatzman touched my head and pushed my hair from my face. His hand was gentle and understanding. A feeling passed between him and me, and a sort of knowing seemed to flow into me from him. I felt at ease. Paul picked me up and carried me out of the room. I was so tired, I just slept for a long time in a deep sleep.

Her recognition in her dream of the anger inside her seemed a step forward. The anger frightened her, but the reassurance she received from Paul and me suggested she was trying to cope with her fear. Since the me of her dream was a creation of her mind, possibly the dream indicated that she was in the process of attempting her own psychotherapy, even while appearing to rely on me.

I met Ruth Thursday evening at the train station, and we went to dinner at an Israeli restaurant near my office.

I was aware that our dining together marked an evolution of our relationship. My role as her psychiatrist or mentor was being replaced by that of her collaborator on a project of mutual interest.

The restaurant was busy and was filled with the noise of customers and the singing of a guitarist.

Ruth asked me about myself for the first time. Why had I chosen to study medicine? Why psychiatry? Was I going to have more children? I answered her questions.

She had never eaten Middle Eastern food before and suggested that I order for her. The questions and answers continued. How did I get on with my parents? Did I have brothers and sisters? And so on.

The waitress leaned over our table to light a candle. I ordered falafel and pita for both of us.

"What do you mainly remember about our first meeting?" Ruth asked. Her question seemed to have romantic implications, however subtle.

"How worried you were," I answered. "And how much you wanted help."

My reply seemed to touch the place in her from which her question had come. "I was sure I was going out of my mind or was already out of it. I'd heard about crazy people being tied up and locked in rooms. I assumed that was how I'd end up."

The guitarist stopped singing to take a break. Ruth lowered her voice. "I remember walking into your office, and as you came in behind me, I was thinking, Where will I start to talk, and after I start, where will it get me? My seeing the apparition of my father had already become a daily event, but I didn't dare tell you about it then. First I had to feel that I could tell you, that you wouldn't put me away. I wanted to trust you. God, how I prayed it wouldn't be a mistake if I did!"

The waitress brought our food. Ruth looked it over. "What's inside the sandwich?" she asked me.

"The brown balls are made of chick peas, there's some salad in there too, and the sauce on the salad is made from sesame seeds."

She took a bite. "What do you think would have happened to me if I hadn't met you?"

"Probably you'd have been referred to another psychiatrist. I guess the psychiatrist would have asked you to enter a mental hospital. It's likely that you'd have been given a drug, maybe two drugs, one to reduce your anxiety and one to relieve your depression. Had a psychiatrist mistakenly considered you schizophrenic, you'd have been given a so-called antischizophrenic drug. I doubt you'd have been locked up, and you certainly wouldn't have been put in a straitjacket. If a psychiatrist had spent time talking to you and learned about the apparition of your father, and if the psychiatrist believed that it's therapeutic to face one's fears, he might have treated you as I did."

"If I hadn't met a psychiatrist like that, what would've become of me in the end?"

"Since your mental health before the crisis had been good, and the crisis came on rapidly, and you were finding your state of mind during it so foreign and so fraught with suffering, you'd have probably emerged from it quickly. Maybe even as quickly as you in fact did."

I was aware that what we were talking about had brought us to reenact the roles of psychiatrist-patient or teacher-student.

After having a few bites of food, she lost interest in it.

"I'm sorry. I just don't feel hungry."

I went on eating, and she sat silently for a moment. "Have you ever seen anyone who wasn't there?" she asked.

"No. Not when awake."

"Heard anyone?"

"No."

"Do you wish you could?"

"Yes, but only if I had some control over it."

"I wish I could teach you how to bring on the experience. But you could teach yourself to, I think, if you wanted to."

"I doubt it."

"Shall I tell you what it's like to do it?"

I nodded.

"Even though it's sometimes hard, it's not like doing a thing with all your might. It's also not a matter of just relaxing and concentrating. It's much more than that."

She looked to see where the waitress was, couldn't see her, turned to me, and asked if she could have a cup of black coffee. "Another thing is that I have to keep my eyes open. I've tried to do it with my eyes closed and I can't."

She looked around again as if to make sure no one was overhearing her, and went on. "So far I've only produced apparitions of people. I tried last night to make an apparition of a dog I'd had as a child, but I couldn't. I've also tried to make a cat, a parrot, and a sunflower, but I couldn't."

"Maybe you could make an apparition of a person who was accompanied by an animal or a flower," I suggested. "And if you then had the apparitional person leave, you might see the animal or flower on its own. If the method worked, you could try it with anything nonhuman."

I glimpsed the waitress and motioned to her. I ordered coffee for Ruth and myself.

"Once this week, while Becky's apparition was visiting me, I tried to write in my diary what was happening. But it was hard to concentrate on keeping her there and to write at the same time."

The coffee arrived, and Ruth sipped it. "Lately I've been finding my concentration also breaks if I speak to an apparition aloud, but not if I speak to it in my imagination."

"How do you talk to it in your imagination?"

"With my thoughts. I don't even have to concentrate. It just knows what's in my mind."

"How does it communicate to you?"

"By speaking or just by thinking. When it speaks, I hear its voice, and see its lips move. But it doesn't need to speak, since I know what it's thinking. There's a connection, a closeness in feeling between it and me."

"When does it speak, and when does it communicate without speaking?"

"There's no rule. It's the apparition's choice at the time."

We finished our coffee. I paid my bill, we left, and I drove her back to her hotel.

We were silent most of the way back.

"What if I wake up tomorrow and I can't make an apparition?" she said playfully, as I dropped her off at the hotel. "What if I can't ever do it again?"

"Is that what you'd like?"

She shrugged her shoulders, laughed, and walked off.

Learning and Limits

I wondered now why I wanted to do our research work.
Was it so that Ruth would learn about herself and
thereby benefit? Was I trying to indulge my scientific curiosity?
To extend human knowledge? Probably all of these, I thought.

She was eager to begin. The only condition she set was that I
explain to her beforehand or afterward the reason for each thing
we would be doing.

As our work would be for the sake of my knowledge as well as
hers, I told her I would stop charging a fee. This did not mean
that her therapy was ended. Within the previous few weeks she
had had some unsettling experiences with apparitions which
indicated she could still use my help. I believed that by exposing
her to the apparitions, our research would increase her mastery of
them and make her stronger.

We spent Friday, Saturday, and Sunday working together, and
the following Thursday, Friday, Saturday, and Sunday. During

these four days I took a hotel room near where she lived, and we spent the time at her home, while Paul looked after the children. After those seven days I did not see her for four weeks. For about two months she had been planning a visit to the United States to see her maternal grandmother, who was terminally ill. The time for that visit had now come.

"I've never produced an apparition of my grandmother and I don't want to, for fear it might harm her," Ruth told me on our first working day. "Maybe I feel that way because my family has told me she's so fragile now, very weak and thin. She's so precious. The only way I want her is in her real form."

"How could you harm her by producing an apparition of her?"

"I don't know. I just don't want to do it. All right?"

"All right."

Once during the seven days that Ruth and I were working together, the grandmother's condition intervened in our research in a remarkable and surprising manner.

In exploring the properties of Ruth's unusual experiences during those seven days, we shuttled back and forth between various lines of inquiry. She could not sustain any of the experiences for more than a few minutes without becoming fatigued. We would stop and chat for a while before resuming work.

On the morning of our first day of work, Ruth and I were in my office.

"Let's do an apparition of me," she said.

"Fine."

She placed an empty chair opposite herself and stared at it intently.

"I see a shadowy figure."

She continued staring. "I feel funny . . . Not uncomfortable, just kind of funny . . . Now I can see her hair and her eyes plainly . . . Now her face . . . She's just sitting there . . . I feel good. I like doing this . . . She's wearing the same ring on her left hand that I'm wearing on my left hand."

That meant that the apparition was not a mirror image of Ruth.

"She doesn't have a bracelet on."

Ruth was wearing a bracelet on her right wrist.

"Actually, I don't like this bracelet. Is that why she doesn't have it on?"

"Could be. Is she sitting like you?"

"Her legs are together, not crossed . . ."

Ruth's legs were crossed.

"And her hands are by her side."

Ruth's hands were on her lap.

"Her clothes?"

"The same as mine." Ruth laughed. "I wonder if our underclothes are the same."

Ruth stared at the chair.

"She's saying, 'Get to know yourself. Ask me questions . . .' When she spoke just then, she gestured in the air. I used to move my hands in the air when I talked, but I got teased about it, so now I don't anymore . . . I feel I could float right into her eyes . . . It's as though she's wanting me to. It's a little spooky . . . Now that I can bring her here, I feel I'll never have trouble remembering anything about myself. I'll just know it all. I guess that sounds corny."

I did not think it corny. I was delighted at the apparition's offer to help Ruth in getting to know herself.

"It's getting hard to hold the apparition here . . . Wait a minute—she's getting up and walking toward the door . . . She's going behind it."

The door to the room was half-open; Ruth was unable to see anything behind it from where she was sitting. The apparition had chosen the only spot in the room where it could hide from her.

Ruth got up to look behind the door.

"I've never followed an apparition before . . . I wonder why she went behind the door . . . She's not there!"

Ruth sat down again. "My head hurts, and my heart is pounding. It's beating all the way up to my throat. I'm not scared, though. It's exciting."

She paused, perhaps to catch her breath. "Could you read your notes back to me?" she said. "I recall only bits and pieces of what went on."

"Is that unusual?"

"I sometimes forget my experiences of an apparition unless I make a particular effort to remember it. That time I was concentrating so hard on her I didn't think to remember."

I read my notes aloud. I reached the part about the apparition getting up and walking behind the door.

"They've got personalities," Ruth commented. "I can't make them do what they don't want to do, or keep them from doing what they want to do. They're like real people. I could say to you, 'Do this,' or 'Don't do that'; you would if you wanted to and wouldn't if you didn't want to."

I recognized, however, that she had gained considerable control over her apparitional experiences since the time her father's apparition had first begun to haunt her.

I finished reading my notes to her.

"When the apparition was sitting down," she added, "I noticed that its legs cast a shadow on the floor."

That gave me an idea for something to try.

Ruth's last remark seemed to have answered the question: Did the apparitions cast shadows? I wanted to confirm that they did. Immediately I thought of another question: If an apparition turned a light on—or off—would Ruth experience a change in the amount of light in the room?

I told her what I was thinking.

She said she would use an apparition of me in trying to resolve my questions.

While she concentrated on bringing into being the apparition of me, I pulled down the window shades and turned out the ceiling light, leaving on a lamp. Then I moved to a position between the lamp and the apparition to find out if I cast a shadow upon the apparition.

She said that I did.

Then the apparition and I changed places with each other.

When the apparition stood between the lamp and me, she saw a shadow fall upon me.

I went over to the lamp and turned it off, so that the only light in the room came through the window shades, which were translucent. I did this to enable her to compare her actually seeing me turn the lamp off with her subsequently hallucinating the same action. After about twenty seconds I put the lamp on again.

She now had the apparition turn the lamp off. She said the amount of light in the room was now the same as when I had in fact turned off the light.

I then actually turned the light off.

She reported no change in the amount of light; she had perfectly hallucinated the darkening of the room.

I asked her to have the apparition put the light on.

She did, and for her the room grew brighter.

When I now actually put the light on, she again saw no change; she had perfectly hallucinated the brightening of the room.

If an apparition turned on a light in a dark room, would Ruth be able to read? If she could, I would be astounded.

I hung thick blankets over the windows and turned off the lamp. I turned off the ceiling light at the wall switch. We sat in the dark for a few minutes so that our eyes could adapt to the dark, but it was still too dark to read. I asked her if she could hallucinate the ceiling light being turned on and then read the name of a book that I would hand to her.

She had an apparition of me turn on the wall switch. She saw the room get lighter, but not as light this time as when the light had actually been on. "It's more of a haze," she said.

Though she could discern the outline of the book's shape—as I could—she could not read its cover.

We repeated the experiment two more times with the same result.

She was deeply disappointed, feeling she had failed.

I reassured her, saying that I hadn't really expected her to succeed, that in the course of learning about her ability, we would no doubt get negative results as well as positive ones, and that a negative result was as useful as a positive one, even if less exciting. Our negative result, moreover, indicated something very important: that apparitions had less power than she did.

I proposed that Ruth try walking around an apparition to see what it looked like from the back.

She said she would create an apparition of Becky. Then Ruth started to circle a spot that was near the center of the room.

"As I'm walking around, she's turning around, so I can't see her back. She's laughing. It's a game she's playing with me . . . Now she's standing still. I can see her back and sides now. She's wearing blue jeans. They look like they've been pressed at the cleaners. She has on a polo sweater and no bra, but that doesn't matter, since she's so flat-chested. And she's wearing clogs, just like a pair I have."

Could Ruth allow herself, I wondered, to be touched by an apparition, or to touch one? If she could, what would it feel like?

"I'll try it," she said, "but I think it'll feel creepy. I'll use an apparition of you. I'll have it sit on the couch next to you."

She stared at a spot to my left for about fifteen seconds. Then she rose from her chair and slowly, cautiously, approached that spot. Timidly she reached out her hand toward the space to my left.

"I'm reaching toward its knees . . . I feel them . . . I don't like it."

"How about trying to hold its hand?"

She shifted her hand a few inches.

"I just touched the top of his hand . . . He didn't mind. But he didn't touch my hand either."

"Touch my hand and compare the feeling."

She did.

"Its hand seems a little colder than yours."

I knew that according to some anecdotes and folklore, an

apparition's touch is often felt as cold. But I didn't know if she knew this.

"Had you expected to find the apparition's hand colder?" I asked.

"I hadn't thought about it."

"Try touching its hand and my hand at the same time, and see if they feel the same or different."

She touched my hand with one hand and its hand with her other hand.

"Its hand seems a little colder, though I'm not sure."

"Does the apparition's hand feel solid, like mine?"

"Yes. If you mean, 'Could I put my hand through it?' the answer is, 'No.'"

"Try the beards."

She touched the apparition's beard and drew her hand back quickly.

"It's beard is prickly . . . I've got the creeps."

"Try again."

She touched my beard with one hand and its beard with the other hand.

"They feel the same."

"Now that you've touched an apparition, could you persuade one to touch you, and maybe to move your body, as the two hospital orderlies lifted you when you were pregnant with Yvonne?"

She was sitting on a chair; a plate with a piece of cake was on her lap.

"I'll try to have an apparition raise one of my legs," she said.

She stretched out her legs onto a nearby footstool, crossing them at the ankles, and held the plate away from her lap.

About fifteen seconds passed. "It's an apparition of you . . . You're leaning over . . . You've got one hand on my heel and the other hand on my calf . . . I feel my leg being raised . . . And now it's being lowered."

As far as I could see, neither of her legs had budged at all.

"Did you see your leg rise?" I asked.

"Yes. Did you?"

"No, not at all."

"I guess when I'd felt myself being lifted off my bed by the orderlies that night, I probably hadn't really been lifted."

I nodded.

"How about having the apparition push down your head from behind?" I suggested. "Let's see whether your head actually moves."

"I'll take the plate off my lap first, so I don't get cake in my face."

She did. About ten seconds passed in silence.

"I can feel the apparition's hand on the back of my head now."

"Who is it an apparition of?"

She turned her head around to look.

"It's you . . . Now it's moving my head down . . . I can see my trousers and part of my blouse right up close."

Her head had moved downward, but only about half an inch.

". . . The hand's gone now. I'm raising my head back up."

As she said that, her head moved upward about the same half an inch.

"My head went all the way down and back up again."

"Can you show me how far?"

She leaned all the way over, so her head was almost in her lap, and then she sat up again.

"When the apparition pushed my head down, what did you see?"

"Your head moved down, but only about half an inch," I replied. "Now you'll never have to fear your father's apparition pushing you in front of a train, because we know your body wouldn't move."

She was silent for a few seconds. "If I allowed an apparition to undress me, would I feel undressed?" she said.

"Why don't you try it some time?"

She blushed. "I've thought of trying to make love with an apparition of Paul," she said.

"Oh?"

"I even mentioned it to Paul last night."

"And?"

"He frowned and grunted. He said, 'All that work with apparitions is getting to you.' I had to laugh."

She continued her account of her talk with Paul. "I said to him, 'It would be a good idea for the time I'll be away visiting my grandmother.'

"He replied, 'The idea makes me jealous.'

"'I wouldn't do it without your consent.' I added, 'But if you won't let me use your apparition, I might use someone else's.' Then he threw a pillow at me.

"I said, 'If I let you know in advance that I was going to do it with your apparition, you could feel good when I did it.'

"He answered, 'But I wouldn't feel it.'

"I don't think he wants me to do it. But I might. I'm so curious." She laughed. "It's not adultery if you make love with an apparition of your husband, is it?"

She didn't wait long to indulge her curiosity. Two days later she told me, "Last night while I was talking to Paul, he fell asleep. He'd kissed me good night, but we hadn't made love. I was feeling a bit lonely for him, so while lying in bed, I produced an apparition of him nude standing beside me. I looked at the apparition for a while. I was feeling bold. The apparition sat down on the bed next to me. He must have read my mind, because he gave me a good old sexy kiss. The kiss was long. He had his hands on either side of my pillow by my head. He pushed my hair back as he always does. Then he caressed my hair, my cheeks, and my chin. I had on a nightgown that was low and loose in front, so that he didn't have to take it off to feel my breasts. I felt so nice and good. Then I asked him to leave. I didn't go any further—honest."

"Did you feel sexually excited?"

"Yeah, just as if it had actually been Paul. My nipples got hard, and my vagina got wet. It's hard for me to believe it happened; I know it wasn't really Paul."

"Have you told Paul?"

"I will eventually."

Once when she was on her own, she made an apparition of me several yards away from her and looked at it through a pair of binoculars.

"As I adjusted the lenses," she said, "it moved in and out of focus just like a person would."

I doubted whether her seeing the figure as being in or out of focus had been dependent upon the focus of the lenses.

"Have you ever seen an image move in and out of focus when you weren't looking at it through binoculars?" I asked.

"Sometimes an apparition will be kind of blurry at first," she said. "Then, as if I've turned a knob, it'll get clearer. That especially happens if I'm doing one apparition right after another."

To explore the matter further, I used a camera which had a range finder.

I stood a few feet from Ruth and measured the distance between us with the range finder. Ruth's face was in focus at a point midway between the 7 and 10 markings, which meant she was about eight and a half feet away.

I then stepped aside and asked her to produce an apparition of me in the very spot I had just been occupying. Meanwhile I passed my fingers over the focusing disc of the range finder, without letting her see whether I was moving the disc or not. I then handed her the camera and asked her to look at the apparition through the range finder and to tell me if it was in focus.

I had moved the disc to the twenty-feet marking.

Ruth looked through the range finder. "The apparition's in focus or almost is," she said.

We did the same experiment five times, each time with the apparition in the same place, eight and a half feet from her. Each time I passed my fingers over the focusing disc, sometimes moving it, sometimes not.

Once, I put the setting midway between the twenty-feet and the infinity markings.

"It's in focus," she said. "If it's out of focus, it's only a little bit."

Would she make the same sorts of mistakes if she looked at a genuine object rather than an apparition? I tested this, and found she did not.

These results suggested that when she had looked at the apparition through binoculars, its passing into and out of focus had occurred without relation to the actual focus of the lenses.

The results also meant—and this is more important—that whatever she was seeing out there was not sending out rays that obeyed the optical laws obeyed by light coming from an actual person.

"I did some experimenting on dope last night," she told me one morning.

"You—dope? You mean—marijuana?"

She nodded. "I smoked it."

"I didn't know you smoke marijuana. Was it the first time?"

She shook her head no. "I used to smoke occasionally, but I haven't for a long while—not unless someone's passing it around at a party. Paul doesn't smoke, so I don't."

"What made you do it this time?"

"I wanted to see how it would affect the apparitions. I did the same apparitions I've done before. They looked like the people they were supposed to look like, but their features were hideous. A face would be elongated with an enlarged forehead, not as much as in a distorting mirror, but enough to be noticeable. On the dope, Paul's apparition had deep lines around its eyes. Afterward I looked at Paul in the flesh and saw the lines, but they weren't as deep. I noticed other features on his face after seeing them exaggerated on his apparition which I hadn't been so aware of before. The same happened with your face. On the dope, I laughed at the faces.

"It was hard to talk to the apparitions, because I found

everything so funny. I'd say to myself, All right, let's look at this experience scientifically. And I'd laugh and say, What's scientifically?—and I'd die laughing.

"The apparitions were in all kinds of crazy places, sitting on top of the television or standing with one leg on the back of a couch and the other leg slung over the banister. The thin wooden supports for the banister didn't bend, but they would've broken if a real person had been standing there. I wasn't consciously putting the apparitions in those places. I was just looking at what they were doing—and laughing. It seemed that everything I saw was funny. I've never thought of doing things like that off dope."

"Sounds as if the apparitions had smoked dope with you," I said.

Earlier I remarked that no apparition that visited Ruth ever left behind it a trace of its visit. Any changes an apparition seemed to make in its environment while it was there disappeared when it did. Ruth had observed this phenomenon many times. Now I wanted to examine the phenomenon once more.

"Why don't you have an apparition write something down?" I said.

"All right."

A pencil and a notebook were lying on the couch. She began to stare at a place on the couch near them. "Oh, my, I don't want that one," she said after a few seconds.

She turned to me. "That was an apparition of my father. I'm not in the mood for him. He's given me a slight headache already."

Again she stared at the place on the couch. "It's an apparition of you," she said. "He's sitting down . . . He's picking up the pencil and paper. The real pencil and paper aren't on the couch now, they're in his hands. What shall I tell him to write?"

"Anything. It doesn't matter what."

"O.K. . . . He's writing now . . . Now he's showing it to me. It's in your handwriting. I can read it plainly. It says, 'Hello, Ruth. This note is to you. Our research is going to interest many people all over the world. Sincerely, Morty Schatzman. . . . I wonder what he means by 'This note is to you.' Is it that the note is only for me? Maybe, because no one else can see it. He's laying the paper down . . . Now he's leaving . . . And now the notebook is back on the couch, and the stupid paper is plain again . . . There's nothing on it."

Given the results of this experiment, I felt virtually certain that a camera would be unable to register an image of an apparition, or a tape recorder its voice. Besides, science and common sense declared such happenings impossible (though some parapsychologists might disagree). Yet I knew that if we tried—and succeeded—the implications would be astonishing, to say the least. There was nothing to lose.

A colleague, Dr. Joseph Berke, who already knew Ruth from her stay at the Crisis Centre, came to my office with his Polaroid camera.

Ruth produced an apparition of me sitting in a chair, and Joe took a picture of the chair. Then I sat in the same chair, and Joe photographed me.

A few moments later, after both pictures had been developed, Joe showed them to her without telling her which picture was of me and which of the apparition.

Ruth saw my photograph in the picture that Joe had taken of me, and saw no figure in the picture that he had taken of the apparition.

Then Joe photographed an empty chair, and the chair with an apparition sitting on it. Ruth tried to say which picture was which, but could see no difference between them.

All our results so far supported Ruth's original view that what she had been seeing was not really there. She was finding it a relief to have this view strengthened.

Our results were consistent, too, with the view that the apparitions were solely a product of Ruth's own mind. Then something happened that made us wonder how firm was the ground we thought we were standing on.

I asked Ruth to have an apparition speak aloud while a tape recorder was on. I wanted to see if she would hear the apparition speaking when the tape was played back.

I told her to signal to me when the apparition began to talk by waving her left hand and to signal when it stopped talking by waving her right hand.

I turned on the tape recorder, and Ruth started to stare at the couch. Almost immediately she waved her left hand. Several seconds later she waved her right hand. Over the course of about ten minutes she signaled altogether four times with each hand; the fourth wave of her right hand was the last signal of the session.

Then Ruth said, "I've got something to tell you, but maybe I shouldn't."

"Is it relevant to our work?"

"Yes. It's also relevant to me . . . That apparition was my grandmother. She appeared before I'd had a chance to concentrate. She's somehow made herself part of our work, though I hadn't wanted her to. She was sitting on the couch, looking pretty.

"She said, 'Cheepy, you already know I need you. I'm waiting for you. And I want to know when you're coming.'

"I was so astonished at hearing her voice that I almost forgot to wave to you at that point.

"Grandma smiled at me. We looked at each other for a long time. She said, 'No matter what happens to me, you'll always have me. I don't want you to worry that you won't. I love you—but you know that. I've done the best I can for you, and you don't owe me anything.'

"I didn't have any thoughts for her to read. I was just feeling kind of sad.

"She began to cry and said, 'I don't want to see you sad.'

"I asked, 'Will I ever see you? Will you be dead when I get home?'

"She replied, 'I'll only be as dead as you'll let me be. Hold your head up, you're as good as the best and better than the rest.' Grandma had tears running down her face, and she was smiling. That was all.

"I hadn't intended to do an apparition of her. But I guess if it just happened and I didn't do it deliberately, there's nothing wrong . . . When she showed up, I thought: She's just died."

Looking at my notes, I saw that the grandmother's apparition had spoken at four separate times. Perhaps these times corresponded with Ruth's four sets of hand-waving signals. I looked at my watch and noted the time—4:41 P.M. I wondered if any crisis had occurred in the grandmother's condition at or around that time.

"If Grandma did die then," Ruth said, "I'll just remember what she told me. Let's keep that part of the tape blank and not play anything else over it."

"I'd like to make sure first that it is in fact blank," I replied. It was; Ruth heard only silence during the replaying of the tape.

"I know there's nothing on it," she said, "but I'd still like to keep it blank. It's of sentimental value to me. I'll write 'Private' on that side of the cassette. I guess you think it's a little stupid to save a tape that doesn't have anything on it."

"I don't. We'll keep it blank. Did that apparition seem different in any way from the others?"

"No, not really. I didn't pay attention to any part of her except her head and shoulders. There is one thing. She looked younger as an apparition than she did when I last saw her—not much younger, because she'd always looked young to me."

Later that day, we again turned the tape recorder on while Ruth had an apparition speak aloud. This time Ruth watched the needle on the tape recorder that indicated recording volume to see if it moved as the apparition was speaking. She found it did not.

"That was Becky's apparition," Ruth said. "She lives near my grandmother and knows my family, so I asked her for information about Grandma.

"The apparition said, 'I'm sorry, Ruth, I don't . . .'—and burst out crying."

The events just recounted took place on a Sunday. Ruth had been scheduled to fly home two days later, early Tuesday morning, to see her grandmother.

On Monday morning Ruth telephoned me at eight.

"I've had some awful news. My mother phoned me at four this morning to say my grandmother died."

"How are you feeling?"

"Terrible. My mother said my grandmother knew I hadn't arrived yet.

"I asked my mother, 'Did Grandma know I was coming?'

"My mother said, 'I told her you were, but I don't know if she understood. She was hallucinating a lot toward the end.' Then, a few hours before she died she said she was going to get some rest. She went into a coma, and never woke up.

"I asked my mother, 'What time did Grandma die?'

"She said, 'A little after five P.M.' That's five P.M. their time, which is eleven P.M. our time.

"I'm still going to fly there tomorrow as scheduled—to the funeral."

About three hours after Ruth had phoned me, I phoned her to find out how she was.

"I've been crying every thirty to forty minutes, just bursting into tears," she said. "In between I've been feeling numb."

At ten in the evening I phoned her again. "I tried to do an apparition of my grandmother today," she said, "but it just didn't work. I tried and I tried, but I couldn't."

"Have you had any other apparitions?"

"No, but I'm pretty sure I haven't lost the ability, in case that's what you were wondering. Just to prove it, I'll do one of you now." She was silent a few seconds. "There, I've done it."

The next morning she flew to her grandmother's hometown.

*   *   *

I was left to puzzle over what had just happened. That visit of the grandmother's apparition fascinated me. It had occurred only six and a half hours before the grandmother's death. It had occurred even nearer in time to—and possibly simultaneously with—the grandmother's entry into her final coma.

Very many anecdotes have been told, I knew, of an apparition of a person manifesting at or near the time of the person's death. For instance, an apparition of Ruth's father's sister, Debbie, allegedly approached her family's home when she had died. I had never come across an interpretation for these asserted coincidences that satisfied me. Could all the testimony be fraudulent? If such coincidences had genuinely occurred, what did they mean?

This was the only time the grandmother's apparition had ever visited Ruth, as far as she could recall. Only a few days before the grandmother had died, Ruth had said that she particularly did not want to create her grandmother's apparition. Its visit, then, was totally unexpected. This in itself would have made me curious. As the apparition's visit was so near in time to the actual death, I felt filled with a sense of the occult.

Meanwhile the voice of orthodoxy was speaking within me: "Suppose Ruth had had no prior inkling that the grandmother was ill; and suppose Ruth had had the same apparitional experience that she in fact did have, and had understood from it (as she in fact did) that her grandmother had died. Then the closeness in time between the apparition's visit and the death would have been striking indeed. However, Ruth had known her grandmother was dying. While she could not have found out by ordinary means the day of the grandmother's death—and she had bought a plane ticket in anticipation of seeing her grandmother alive—she had been expecting the death soon. This consideration makes the coincidence between the two events less remarkable. Her grand-mother's apparition, like the other apparitions, could have been produced solely by Ruth's creative mental faculties. Its manifesta-tion could have been expressing Ruth's guess about the time of her grandmother's death—a sudden, impulsive, and unconsciously formulated guess, but an informed one. That is the only clear and plausible interpretation of the coincidence."

Another voice followed this one, chiming in with, "Suppose the apparition had delivered news of the manner of the grandmother's death, and suppose Ruth had later found the news to be correct. That too would have been striking." However, the apparition had not done that.

A third voice joined in, saying, "According to Ruth, the mother said that the grandmother 'was hallucinating a lot toward the end.' Suppose the grandmother had described seeing or hearing Ruth, and suppose her description had later been found to match Ruth's actual appearance, behavior, or circumstances that day. That too . . . But here again evidence is lacking."

My verdict on the matter was that it was suggestive, mysterious, even tantalizing, but inconclusive. If only I would see a way to investigate further . . . but I could not.

Daughter and "Father"

WHILE the events just recounted were occurring, Ruth discovered that she could create her father's face upon her own face as she looked into a mirror. She had already seen his face appear upon my face and upon Yvonne's and Paul's faces. Now, in my presence, she looked at herself in a mirror and changed the image of her reflected face into an image of her father's face.

She and I had first discussed this experiment in one of our early-morning telephone talks. We hoped that it might teach us something about her, her father, and their relationship. She had said she would like to try it if I was with her at the time. We did this experiment eight times before she left for her grandmother's funeral.

Ruth called this project "the weirdest thing we've done." I found it most interesting and unusual, and during it I witnessed events of a sort that were new in my experience. My relation with Ruth until now had been impressing upon me that the human understanding of the mind is very limited and that much indeed remains unknown. What I now observed impressed that awareness on me even more.

The first time she set about it, she sat on the floor and asked me to sit on a chair behind her and near her. That way she could see my reflection in the mirror if she needed to. It was for her "security," she said. If her father's face appeared to replace her face, then her father might "take over" her being—in which case she wanted me to be nearby.

I was to address questions to the person occupying her body, she said. She wanted me to try to find out from that person why her father had left the family when she was six weeks old, why he had later returned, and why he had assaulted her when she was ten. She expected the answers would be voiced by her vocal cords and would come from her mouth.

What was next said I wrote down verbatim while sitting behind her. After her experience had ended and we had discussed it, I read my notes to her, which she commented upon. She felt that some of the words which had emerged from her mouth earlier had been spoken by her, but that most had been spoken by her father. The following transcript keeps to her indications about who said what. I enclose "father" within quotation marks, as I am uncertain what status to grant to the entity which she alleges was her father and which spoke through her mouth. Some of her subsequent comments appear in brackets.

RUTH: Here I go, Dr. Schatzman. . . . I don't know if it's going to work. (*She is sitting, staring at her reflection in the mirror.*) I can see him in the mirror perfectly . . . I still feel I'm me, but that feeling is changing.

I: Who are you now?

"FATHER": You tell me. (*The "father" is visibly trembling.*)

I: What are you doing here?

"FATHER": I'm visiting. Why? (*The trembling increases.*)

RUTH: I don't want to do this. . . .

[Ruth later told me that she had not wanted to go on

at this point. She said she hadn't wanted to, "because feeling his feelings so strongly frightened me. It made me feel part of him. I wanted to be separate from him, to be farther away from him. But I'd still been curious to see what would happen."] No, Dr. Schatzman. Keep on.

I: And now, who are you?

"FATHER": What's it to you?

I: I'm interested for Ruth's sake more than mine.

"FATHER": Sometimes I love her. Sometimes I despise her, the little bitch.

I: Why do you sometimes despise her?

"FATHER": She rejected me.

I: Are you referring to the time you tried to have intercourse with her?

"FATHER": She rejected me before then. I always wanted to touch her. *(The "father" clasps a hand to his chest and takes a deep breath.)* I've always wanted to love her. I wouldn't have hurt her.

I: Why were you more interested in her than in Mallory?

"FATHER": Why are you interested in me?

I: Mainly because I want to understand Ruth.

"FATHER": She was more affectionate than Mallory. She'd get on my lap and tell me she wanted to talk about the stars. *(The "father" laughs lewdly.)* I knew she wanted it. She wanted it like the rest of them wanted it.
[Ruth told me afterward she recalled him wanting her to love him when she was a child. She was sure a sexual interpretation of why she sat on his lap was mistaken.]

I: Why did you leave her and the family when she was six weeks old?

"FATHER": I had to go. The law was after me for hot checks.
[Ruth later told me that she had once heard this is why he had left, but she had never been certain if it was true.]

I: Where did you go?

"FATHER": To New York. Then I caught a train to Canada. I was away long enough and came back. They brought me back.

I: Who did?

"FATHER": The police.

I: And then?

"FATHER": I did time in jail. I was released on parole. I went to Oregon.

I: What did you do there?

"FATHER": Factory work.

I: Then what happened?

"FATHER": I wrote to Sue [Ruth's mother] and sent the kids presents.

RUTH: Dr. Schatzman, I'm getting sick.

I: Do you want to stop?

RUTH: No. No, let's go on.

I: What happened next?

"FATHER": Sue wrote and said she'd received the presents. I decided to visit and that's when I met her.

[Ruth explained to me that in real life her father often referred to her as "her" and "she" instead of by name.]

I: How old was Ruth then?

"FATHER": A little bitty thing. I knew Sue had been messing with other men, so I left. One was a weasel of a man.

[Ruth recalled that she liked that man and that the man had liked her mother and the children, but that her mother had refused to marry him.]

I went back to Oregon. Caught a freight, bummed around, went South, went back North. Sue and I tried to patch it up. I really tried.

I: And how did things go with Ruth?

"FATHER": She loved me right off. Mallory was something else. She cried and begged her mother not to take me

back. Ol' Sue came across though. I knew she'd take
me back.

RUTH: Dr. Schatzman, hurry. I'm getting sick.

I: Do you remember the night of your sexual attack upon
Ruth?

"FATHER": She was warm and tiny. *(The "father" is shaking
now and breathing heavily.)* She said she loved me. I
wasn't going to hurt her.

RUTH: Dr. Schatzman, hold on to me. This is scary.
[Afterward she said that here she was aware of "his"
feelings more than at any other time. She felt "him"
to be very angry and violent, and she felt frightened.]

"FATHER": I wanted her to bleed. She was so warm. She's
always warm. If I started up again with her now,
she'd stay with me always. *(The "father" is breathing
heavily.)*

RUTH: Why don't we stop?

Throughout this experience, even when calling to me, she
stared at the mirror, her gaze never wavering. The voice and
intonation with which words were spoken, whether by her or by
her "father," were hers. When her "father" was speaking, her
face seemed expressionless, masklike, and stiff, in a way that I
found uncharacteristic of her. As I had never actually met her
father, I did not know if his face was like this.

When her experience had ended, she said to me, "That was
terrible. I've got a pounding headache. My chest hurts. My face is
burning. I feel nauseous. It was hard not to vomit, but I thought
it was important to go on. I feel pins and needles all over, as if my
body had been asleep."

I felt her wrist pulse; it was beating strongly at a rate of one
hundred beats a minute.

"I didn't lose touch with myself," she continued. "He didn't
take over my body. I was feeling his feelings, which frightened
me. But the feeling of being frightened was my own. I was feeling

my own feelings as well as his. I'm not too frightened now that it's over . . . He doesn't like you—or me."

I knew that many psychotherapists believe that experiencing strong emotions in the therapist's presence is therapeutic. If they are right, then Ruth was being benefited, and perhaps her "father" was too.

"Do you recall what he said?" I asked.

"Vaguely. Let's see what I remember . . . You asked him what he was doing here. I can't call to mind what he said. And you asked him when he'd first seen me. Usually when I remember my first meeting with him, I see him there, standing on the sidewalk. But just now, it was myself I saw there, as if through his eyes. I had on a pair of blue shorts and a top that was just a little stretchy band, and I was barefoot with dirty feet . . . For those moments I was there, reliving that meeting. But it seems as though I had his memory of me, not my memory of him. I know now exactly how he'd felt then. He'd been afraid."

Ruth's recall of the experience she had just undergone was incomplete and poorer than of many of her apparitional experiences. Perhaps this signified a difference between her mental state in this experience and in the other experiences.

"Besides fear, did you notice any other feelings he had toward you?"

"Anger and sexual desire. His sex urge was stronger than any I've ever felt. He had to do what he did. He didn't have any control. I'm going to tell you something now that will amaze you. My panties are wet, and I think it's from sexual excitement. They got wet during the part about the rape."

At first I assumed it was the "father" who had become sexually excited, not Ruth at ten years old or Ruth now—though later I was to reconsider. If it was the "father," then her fear that he might take over her body seemed to have been fulfilled. But can one say that Ruth was taken over or possessed if she had brought on the experience voluntarily?

The information about the father's past given here by the "father" raised two further questions. Was the information true?

Had Ruth already possessed the information before the trance? I could only pose the questions; I could not answer them satisfactorily. She did not know whether the information was true. Further, she did not know whether she had already heard the information from others in her family, and she didn't want to ask them. She had not told her family about her recent emotional crisis or about her work with me, and did not wish to give them the slightest grounds for suspecting what she had been involved in. Some of the information seemed completely new to her. It is very difficult to rule out the possibility that one has heard something and forgotten it. I was certain she had never before told me the information that she regarded as new. I believed the most plausible interpretation of what had happened was that the "father" had been reporting here information Ruth had once known, but had forgotten.

In trying to understand the form of Ruth's experience, I considered an analogy with acting and role-playing. While onstage, some actors and actresses are aware of themselves as persons playing the parts of other persons, and of the differences between those others' personalities and their own offstage selves. But some actors and actresses lose themselves in their roles so completely that they become largely unaware of the audience, the theater, and even themselves as distinct from the roles they are playing. Perhaps Ruth had been immersed in playing the role of her father—immersed enough to get sexually excited, but not so immersed as to lose all awareness of her own feelings or to imitate her father's voice.

I also saw a similarity between Ruth's experience and what I knew about trance mediumship. C. D. Broad, a Cambridge philosopher, has described some typical phenomena of trance mediumship. As most eminent trance mediums in Western countries in the past 150 years have been women, he refers to the medium as "she":

> When a trance-medium is about to give a sitting to a client, she generally begins by shutting her eyes while resting

quietly in her chair. Soon after this she begins to breathe deeply, to groan slightly and to struggle, and in general to behave like a person who is profoundly but restlessly asleep and is suffering from a rather distressing dream. In a few minutes, as a rule, she becomes calmer, and one often hears a kind of whispering going on, as if she were talking to herself. Shortly after this she will begin to talk audibly, often in a very different voice and manner and sometimes with a very different vocabulary from those which are characteristic of her normal waking conversation. Ostensibly the medium's normal waking personality has ceased to control her vocal organs, and a new personality has gained control of them.

The new personality may carry on a conversation with the sitter for an hour or more. Eventually it says that it must leave, and it bids the sitter good-bye. The process with which the sitting began is then repeated in the reverse order. In a few minutes, after a certain amount of struggling, groaning, and whispering, the eyes are again opened, and the medium resumes her normal voice and manner. She is generally ignorant of what has been happening during the sitting; just as a person who has been talking in his sleep is ignorant of what he has been doing and saying, and rapidly forgets what he has been dreaming, when he awakes. On the other hand, the trance-personality often claims to be aware of what was being done and perceived and thought by the medium at times when the normal personality was in control of the body and the trance-personality was in abeyance. . . .[16]

Ruth's experience resembled in two ways the trance described. Firstly, she seemed to talk with me in the person of someone other than herself. Secondly, immediately after her experience ended, she was largely ignorant of much that had gone on during it. In other respects her experience differed from the one quoted.

I shall refer to this particular experience Ruth had—and to others she subsequently had of the same type—as a trance. In using this term I am not suggesting that I understand her experiences. Nor am I implying that her experiences of apparitions occurred in a state that could not also be called a trance. I am using the term merely as a convenience to indicate the special sort of experience she had that I have just narrated.

The next morning we began as before, she sitting on the floor in front of a full-length mirror and I sitting behind her with a notepad.

She later said that this time, instead of trying to see her father's face in the mirror, she imagined his face. "That's all I had to do, and my face started changing into his. Suddenly there were his eyes, and nose, and graying hair on the sides of the face, and balding head. I didn't pay attention to the body, just the face . . . I decided to try very hard to stay aware of all his feelings, so I could answer your questions later, and to feel what he was feeling."

Again, inserted in brackets are her comments about the trance after she emerged from it.

> RUTH (she is staring at the mirror): I can feel a feeling. He's scared. He's sorry he did something.
>
> I: What did he do?
>
> RUTH: Somehow I think they were involved. He loves her a lot, more than anyone else, I think. I know his love isn't exactly like a brother's. (Ruth is trembling.) She gave him drugs first, before he ever took any. They took them together. [Ruth later explained she was referring here to her father's relation with Debbie, his sister who had died at seventeen. "At this point in the experience my father was thinking about Debbie's beautiful body, about her long, slim, pretty legs. What did go on between him and her? I think she's the reason he hasn't been able to love my mother more . . . My mother told me Debbie had been beautiful. I know my mother got information about her from my father's mother. I wonder why my mother has been so

interested in Debbie . . . To me Debbie has always been a mystery."]

I: Can you say any more about the circumstances of Debbie's death?

RUTH: No . . . Dr. Schatzman, is this eye, my right eye, different from the other one?

I: Yes, your right eyelid is a little lower than the left one. Why do you ask?

RUTH: One of his eyes doesn't open as wide as the other when he's been drinking.

I: Hmmmm. Yesterday you were feeling his feelings in relation to the rape. Can we return to that? [She said later that, at this moment, "I saw him coming into my bedroom, looking like he looked then—not over-weight like he is now. I was seeing the scene from my bed."]

RUTH: He's in bed with me. (*Ruth—or the "father"—is breathing deeply and staring at the mirror.*) He wants to take my panties off. He wants to feel her—should I say the word?—pussy. He tries to get his finger in, but the pussy isn't wet. He tries to lick it, she's fighting him, kicking him, which makes him mad. He slaps me and says I'd better be still.

[Afterward, I pointed out to Ruth that she had sometimes referred here to the little girl as "I" and "me," and sometimes as "she" and "her." Ruth explained that she had been simultaneously aware of the girl's experience from within, as if it had been her own experience, and of the girl's behavior from without, as if she had been a separate person.]

He puts his hands on the insides of the tops of my legs. It feels like they're going to break. He's taking his penis and trying to get it in, but it won't go in. He's holding it and thinking where he can put it in. He's struggling to hold me down. He's trying to put it in my armpit. I'm on my tummy now. He's thinking

my rectum might be bigger. He's mad—more than
mad—desperate. He's got my head. My head is all
pounding. He's sitting on me and pulling on my hair,
jerking it. He's trying to get his penis into my mouth.
I can taste it. He's about to climax. He just did. I'm
crying and shaking inside. (*Ruth—or the "father"—is
sitting staring at the mirror, not moving and breathing
hard.*)
　　He wants to know if I'm in pain. He tells me if I
hadn't fought he wouldn't have hurt me. He says I'd
better not tell my mother. He swears he'll kill me if I
do. I'm thinking I'll tell her. He's thinking my mother
won't believe me.
　　He's putting his underwear in with the dirty
clothes. He's going to take a bath. I think he's
whistling.
　　I feel pain when I move my legs. There's blood on
my chest, and my nipples burn and hurt.

At this point Ruth's face abruptly relaxed—and the trance was
over.
　　"All he was thinking about was getting his penis inside me. He
wasn't bothered about hitting me and biting me. He had no
thought of how small I was. I know because I was thinking his
thoughts. I believe he may have penetrated me a little bit. When
he started building up to a climax, he got desperate again, wanting
to be inside me. It wasn't making love he wanted. He just wanted
to get it inside whatever opening he could. When he finally did
climax, he was using his hand on his penis, holding it next to my
face and jerking it all over me like a hose. At the moment of his
climax, I could feel his enjoyment. Hitting me and climaxing at
the same time made it wonderful for him. Is it possible that
hurting me was part of his enjoyment?"
　　"Yes," I replied.
　　"I got wet in my pants again today."
　　I said nothing.

"I don't think he felt any guilt. When he was through he felt just like he always feels, except in a better mood. For him, it was over and he wanted to sleep.

"One of my nipples still has a scar. When I breast-fed, that breast hurt. I couldn't stay on it long and had to change to the other one.

"Another thing: I didn't look at your reflection at all that time. But I felt your presence with me. At one point I felt a need to reach up and take your hand, but I didn't."

How was I to understand Ruth's awareness of herself from both the child's viewpoint, as if Ruth had been reliving the experience, and from an outside observer's, as if she had been watching the child? I did not know, but I reflected that many people's memories of early childhood experiences, including mine, often have the same peculiar feature. Ruth's experience did not seem unusual in this regard.

What did seem unusual was that much of the experience had been undergone from the father's point of view. This had been so, she said afterward, despite her having referred to him throughout as "he" and "him," not as "I" and "me." She said, "I could feel for him as well as for myself. I'm sure I was feeling his feelings much of the time." At various moments she had reported his feelings as if she had been privy to them, for example the pounding in his head while he attacked her.

I hoped that in the course of thinking the thoughts and feeling the feelings of her "father," she would be able to gain more understanding of her actual father and of herself. Perhaps, as a result, she would become less fearful of her father.

I considered her account of the assault remarkably vivid and dramatic. She had portrayed not only what the child, or someone else in the room at that time, might have seen or heard, but also what that child had apparently tasted—the father's penis in her mouth—and felt—pain when she moved her legs, and burning and hurt in her nipples. Ruth's use throughout of the present tense had made it seem as if she had been having the experience for the first time.

I was fascinated with what had been unfolding before my eyes. I decided I would try to comprehend it more fully.

Although it had been an ordeal, Ruth was soon ready to try once more.

"This time I'm going to try not to see my face at all—only his—to let go more, to try to go completely into his feelings. But you have to take care of me."

She assumed her usual position, as I did. She was staring at the mirror.

RUTH: My forehead is smooth. I'm bald. My eyebrows are real bushy. My eyes are sparkling. The eyeballs are red. All right, I have all my father's features . . . I can feel his feelings. They're stronger than my feelings. I'm going to see if I can feel them even stronger.

I: What was meant the other day at the end of the trance by "I wanted her to bleed"?

"FATHER": I wanted her to bleed over me. I want to screw her so good—and stay inside.

I: Why do you want her to bleed over you?

"FATHER": It would be warm. And it would bleed into me. I'd be hers.

I: What do you mean?

"FATHER": I'd be safe. I don't know. I've got to do it, be inside her, to be inside each drop of blood . . . I want to be all inside, to crawl up inside of her, her pussy, her stomach, and her ass.

I: Have you wanted to be her baby?

"FATHER": She had a baby, a little girl. I thought about that baby coming out. She was empty then. It was good there, safe and warm. I wanted to get in her then. I wanted to suck her breast.

I: But you've never been inside Ruth. Who are you talking about?

"FATHER": I'm talking about Ruth. She wouldn't let me get in. She fought me and screamed. I didn't want to hurt her at first. I just wanted to get in . . . I want to kill her. Oh, I hate her. I've got to be there. I want to see her bleed. *(The "father" is breathing hard with fists clenched, staring straight ahead.)*

I: Bleed from where?

"FATHER": From her pussy and her ass.

I: Why from there?

"FATHER": Because then I can get in. It's got to be as small a place as I can get into—so I can't come out.

I: How would her bleeding help you?

"FATHER": I'm not sure. It's just got to be like that. After that I don't care what would happen to me. I'd put my face in first and climb in.

I: What are you looking for in there?

"FATHER": If I get in, I'll stay and never come back out.

I: Why choose Ruth?

"FATHER": She's tiny and lovely and sweet. I'd have her all around me . . . I want to be in her and in the blood. I want to be deep in her, as deep as deep can be. I want her to close up all around me. Just soft. I don't want any air or light to get in.

I: You know, it sounds to me like you might want to die inside Ruth. But what's special about her?

"FATHER": Oh, God, I love her. I just want to love her. It's all right, you know. It's not like loving Mallory. It's different with Ruth. I just want to kiss her and hold her.

RUTH: Dr. Schatzman, I'm getting tired. I feel faint. *(Ruth buries her head in her hands.)* I'm sorry, I just can't do it any longer. What's happening? How long have you talked with me?

She was now out of the trance.

"I went faint," she said. "Everything went black—so I put my head down. That's what everyone says to do . . . At that point my vision blurred, and I lost touch with my father."

I read back my notes of the session.

A few times she winced, especially when I read the parts about crawling up inside her "pussy" and her "ass" and bleeding from her "pussy" and her "ass." These words were not the sort she ordinarily used. She seemed discomforted that they had come from her mouth.

When I'd finished reading, she said, "I lost all contact with everything about myself, with all that I'm familiar with except your voice. All I was conscious of was his face and your voice."

"What do you make of what was said in the session?"

"With a father like that I might not have made it in life if it hadn't been for my grandmother's love."

"Have you ever thought before just now that your father's mind might have worked in the way we've just heard?"

"No. It sounded very strange to me."

"I wonder if the talk about getting deep inside you is connected with the attack happening on the night after your mother delivered Jane."

"I'm not sure I understand."

"I'll read from my notes. 'She had a baby, a little girl.' In fact, your mother had just had a baby girl. I'm reading from my notes again. 'I thought about that baby coming out. She was empty then. It was good there, safe and warm. I wanted to get in her then. I wanted to suck her breast.' If those thoughts had really been your father's, then his having wanted to put his penis into your vagina could mean that he'd been confusing your womb with your mother's womb, and perhaps even confusing his penis with a baby."

Ruth nodded and said nothing.

I knew that the connection I had just put forth was plausible psychologically. It was especially plausible given Ruth's allegation that a doctor had once labeled the father schizophrenic—though based on what I knew of the father, I believed many psychiatrists might have called him a borderline schizophrenic or a severe personality disorder. The sort of person who warrants any of these labels might well be confused in the way that the "father" of her trances seemed to have been. All her utterances just now in the person of the "father" were consistent with the thinking of a man who might try to rape his young daughter on the night after his wife had delivered a baby. I was intrigued, because Ruth had never before indicated insight into why her father had attacked her, or why he had done so on that particular night. Nor had she ever expressed to me the sort of thinking that characterizes people with schizophrenia, borderline schizophrenia, or a severe personality disorder.

What then, I wondered, was the source of the statements in this trance? Might the "father" have been repeating here remarks of a sort Ruth had once heard her actual father make? Perhaps so, but she could not recall ever having heard him say such things.

The next time we tried a trance, I decided to deal with other matters.

It began in the usual way, in front of the mirror.

"My nose is bigger, my face is red. O.K., I'm looking like him . . . I'm beginning to feel like he does. I can feel my feelings, but not so much now. I feel his feelings stronger . . . His feelings are almost all the feelings now. O.K. What do you want to know?"

I: How did you feel about Ruth when she was a child?

"FATHER": She wouldn't talk to me. She didn't act like a little girl should act. She'd never stay in and help her mother. She stayed with boys playing ball—so she said. (*The "father" laughs lewdly.*)

I: Why are you laughing?

"FATHER": I know what she was doing with them. So do you.

I: What was that?

"FATHER": Teasing them—like she teased me. The little bitch!

I: Why did you shoot at her?

"FATHER": I hate her. She's laughing at me. I see the way
she looks at me when she walks into the room. She
loves me, and then she runs away from me and laughs
at me. You goddamned little motherfucking whore
bastard, I'll kill you.

I: What's she laughing at you for?

"FATHER": She knows.

I: Why do you want to kill her?

RUTH: He's afraid I'm going to hurt him. I'm a threat.

I: Why do you want to shoot her?

"FATHER": I don't. I missed.

I: You missed purposely?

"FATHER": No. I just hate her. She won't love me. (*Heavy
breathing.*) She's a vicious, spiteful little girl. She's
already a whore. You have to watch her and see her
outside. I watch her. Those little shorts. She has to
have them up to her ass or she won't wear them. I'll
rip them to hell. I'll kill her. I'll bide my time and by
God I'll get her. She won't laugh at me again. I know
she'll fuck anyone behind my back. Why won't she
give me one little screw, just one? She wouldn't even
miss it. (*Lewd laughter.*) How could it hurt her? All
it would do would be to make me feel good. Then
she'd love me and she'd never leave me, and I'd be her
baby. . . .

She knows things about me. She saw me. She
shouldn't have come back in. I told her to stay
outside. If she tells Sue, Sue will leave me. I'll have
nowhere to stay. I'll be cold and hungry . . . Screwing
little nigger girls ain't wrong . . . She just saw me.
She ran. I've got to catch her before she gets back to
the house.

I: Who is "she"?

"FATHER": Ruth. She must have come in the back way. I've
got to catch her. Where did she go? Goddamn. She
went to those woods. I'll get her some candy.

RUTH: Dr. Schatzman, my head is hurting. I'm dizzy. Am I going to faint? I don't think I can get up.

The trance was over. In a few moments Ruth had recovered.

I asked, "What was that last bit about when your father said you knew things about him, when he said, 'She saw me. She shouldn't have come back in,' and all the rest?"

"There was a shed across the street from our house. An old couch was in there that we'd jump up and down and play on. One day—I was about eight—no one was around, so I decided to go play there.

"I went around to the back. I heard a little girl crying. I pushed open the door. My father had that little girl lying on the couch. She was about my age. He was pushing his penis in and out. She didn't seem to like it. I'm not sure if I knew then what he was doing, but I knew it was wrong. I was so disappointed, because I'd thought I finally had a really good daddy.

"I ran, and kept on running. I stubbed my toe. It hurt. I went way down into the woods where no one goes, and I just sat there for a long time. I was afraid to go home. I hid and watched the house.

"When I saw my mama go in, I slipped in behind her. I went up to my room. He came to the door of my room and just looked at me. I didn't say anything. I just looked back at him.

"I never did see that little girl again. She was black. She had lots of pigtails all over her head and a ribbon in her hair. I wonder what happened to her. I've never told anyone about it."

I asked, "How come you never told me?"

"I'd forgotten it. I don't think I ever dared remember it. Probably I was afraid of what my father would do if I did remember it. Also, I was so disappointed in him. It was as if he'd broken my heart. I'd rather it had stayed buried. I'm trying hard not to cry. I wonder how many other girls he did that to . . . There's probably another reason I forgot it: I needed to keep my sanity.

"The more I go into this," she said, "the less I hate him, and the more I feel sorry for him and want to help him."

Ruth's experiences of her "father" were producing empathy in her for her actual father.

If this incident with the black girl had truly happened, and Ruth had forgotten it, her forgetting had been self-serving and had possibly been illustrating more a skill for putting the thing out of her mind than a memory failure.

The "father" brought up this event just after asserting that Ruth would "fuck anyone behind my back." Yet "he" had apparently been doing it behind someone's back—"his" wife's. The "father," then, was seeing in Ruth a tendency which appeared to correspond with "his" own behavior. Similarly, the "father" assumed Ruth had been involved in sexual acts with children (though she had not, as far as I knew), when "he," apparently, was the one who desired children sexually. "He" was attributing inclinations to her that on the face of it were "his." "He" was thereby displaying the mechanism of paranoid projection; that is to say, "he" seemed to be attributing to her an aspect of "his" own disposition, and was feeling persecuted by that aspect. Here again a psychologically plausible picture of disordered thinking was emerging, this time with a paranoid flavor.

The "father" was speaking as if the feelings and events being cited were present here and now. For instance, "he" was saying that if Ruth tells Sue what "he" has been up to, Sue *"will"* leave him; this is how the father might have put it at the time the incident actually happened, seventeen years earlier.

The next time we did the exercise I wanted to pursue further the matter of the father's shooting at Ruth.

"I'd feel more comfortable if there were less light," she said when we began. "I'd feel more relaxed and I'd get into the experience more easily."

I drew the curtains. It was still light enough for her to see her reflection in the mirror.

She stared for a few moments at the mirror and tensed her fingers tightly as if they were clasping something.

RUTH: O.K., I can see him. I can feel him, but I can feel myself as well . . . I'm out of him a little bit, but if you wait a few seconds, I'll be in, and then it will be just him speaking. *(The fingers tensed more tightly.)*

I: *(I waited about thirty seconds.)* Do you recall the time you shot at Ruth?

"FATHER": I see her sitting on a couch. The couch is against the wall. There are purple drapes.

I: What else?

"FATHER": Sue is in the kitchen frying potatoes. She's arguing with me about me coming home drunk, and me spending money. I haven't paid the electricity bill. She says, "You're causing Ruth to be upset. You should be quiet." I say, "It's my house." Ruth is staring at me. She seems to be staring through me. She always does this. She's vicious and spiteful.

I: Then what happens?

"FATHER": I ask her, "What in hell are you looking at?" She says, "Nothing, Daddy." I say, "You goddamned little bitch, am I nothing?" She's got her goddamned little nose up in the air. She thinks she's better than all of us. I know her. I despise the little bitch. Do you know what it's like to despise someone so much and you can't do anything about it? She's got a way. She can make me love her one minute, and hate her the next.

I wanted to kill her. The very last minute maybe I didn't want to. I missed, and I didn't want to miss. I never miss. I'm a good shot. I could hit a squirrel on a tree. She screamed, and put her hands over her ears and ran.

[Ruth said later that at this point she saw herself, through his eyes, leave the house by the front door, and also actually heard the screen door slam.]

I'm trying to get another shell into the gun.

She'll call the cops. I'll kill her if she does. Oh,
God, I don't want them to take me. I don't want to be
locked up. The goddamned little bitch. I'll leave. No,
I'll lock the doors. They've got to have a warrant to get
in. Goddamn, I shouldn't have missed. I wanted to
get rid of her once and for all. But I got confused.

They're hurting my arm. That bastard cop is doing
it on purpose. Goddamn it. Oh, God, I'll do anything.
Just don't lock me up.

I: What happened next?

"FATHER": I went before the judge: "Disturbing the peace.
Drunk and disorderly conduct." I pleaded guilty.

I'll get her. I'll get her. We could be happy if she
wouldn't keep on. I don't want to go home if she is
there. I don't want to go back to that motherfucking
house if she's there. I can't stand it. All I have to do is
look at her, and I want to kill her. I can't stand it. I
don't want to hate her. I hate to see anyone hurt her.
But that's when she's being very good. I can't make
her understand.

Sue got her a training bra. Ha! I looked at it and I
wanted to squeeze her tits so badly.

RUTH: Dr. Schatzman, it's getting harder. I'm trying hard. I
see him now, but I don't think I'll be able to see him
much longer. His beard is getting lighter.

She buried her face in her hands, and the trance ended.

I asked, "How are you feeling?"

"Exhausted. But not as bad as I felt the last time I did him. Let
me tell you about what goes on in these experiences. I have to
concentrate on relaxing, and not holding on to my feelings. When
I do that, first I feel my heart beating fast. I feel scared. It's like
another feeling starts pushing my feelings out. And the next thing
I know, I'm not aware of what's around me—at least, I think
that's what happens."

"What are you seeing during the experience?"

"Before I start, I look at the mirror and see myself. Then I see him, just him. At the point that I'm having my feelings and his at the same time, I'm seeing him, not me. This time when I saw him, he looked about fifteen years younger than he's looked as an apparition."

"What do you remember of the trance experience?"

"I recall it all up to the point where you asked about the shooting. I was concentrating on his feelings, not on mine. I can't remember anything after I started to feel his feelings. If you gave me a pen and paper, and said my life depends on remembering, I couldn't. It's just gone."

I now read back to her my notes of the session.

When I'd finished, she said, "During the first part, I remember I was trying to hold on to his feelings. I was no longer seeing this room; I was seeing that room. I was seeing the couch and the purple drapes—I'd forgotten those drapes. He was the one doing the looking. He was seeing me sitting on the couch as a little girl with long hair. Since I'd cut it just after the rape, the shooting must have happened before the rape."

"How do you understand his talking to me in these sessions? Does he know it's me?"

"I don't see how he could; he doesn't know you. But he's answering you, which means he's talking to you. I don't know. While you're reading it back to me, it's vaguely familiar. It never surprises me. It might scare me, but it doesn't surprise me.

"It's so close to me. I remember my feelings from the time these things originally happened. When I was staring at him then, I was in the living room. He'd just come out of the kitchen. He thought that I was staring at him to be rude or that I was a witch, but I think I was just afraid of him. I was only trying to keep out of his way. When he was in that state, it seemed I couldn't keep out of his way.

"Another thing: I don't think I called the cops that time. I wasn't in any condition to. Someone else did. I'd called them other times. I wonder why he didn't know they'd come and get him. Why did he do it if he was so afraid of the cops? Maybe he wasn't afraid of them, but of going to the mental hospital. When the cops came and he was about to go, I think he felt like crying. He was feeling lost, and in despair."

I said to Ruth, "Do you think if I'd asked you yesterday in your normal state to recall that shooting event in detail, you would have been able to recall as much as you have?"

"I don't think so. For instance, I don't believe I'd have remembered the part about my mother and him fighting over the electricity bill."

She paused and took a deep breath. "You know," she said, "the more we do this, and the more we learn about that old rascal, the more I pity him. He thinks that other people are crazy, and that he's fine. I understand now a little about how he felt, about how I've been someone he's resented, hated, and feared.

"When I go home, I'm going to try to get to know him. I don't mean I'm going to risk my life. I'm not going to let him touch me or maul me. If there were any possibility—which I doubt—I'd even like to help him. But I don't begin to know how. And you can't help someone you're afraid of."

A few days later, I suggested we try the exercise again.

Ruth said, "I did one of these at home this week. I can't remember what happened during it. I can become him easily now. I can do it without a mirror. I make an apparition of him, and then the apparition and I approach each other. We come closer and closer together until we merge with each other."

"Why don't you try it that way now?"

She was sitting in a chair.

"O.K. Give me about twenty seconds to get deep into it."

She clenched her hands.

The next words that were spoken came from her mouth: "I'm here."

"Who is?" I asked. "Who's here?"

"A. C. Sergeant." It was Ruth's father's name.

"How do you feel about the fact that you'll soon be seeing Ruth?"

"I'll be glad to see her."

"Do you think about her?"

"Just about every day."

"What are your thoughts when you think about her?"

"I wonder what she's doing and how she's doing. I miss her. Me and her don't get along too well. She can be vicious, but she's tenderhearted. I know her better than I know anyone else in the world."

Ruth's face was virtually expressionless, just as it had been when we'd done the exercise in front of the mirror. She looked at me throughout the conversation with a blank stare.

"How do you think she's feeling toward you?" I asked.

"She doesn't like me too much. But she comes across if I need her. Blood is thicker than water."

"How are you feeling these days about what she says you did to her when she was ten?"

"That's a damned lie. She made it up."

"You and I talked about it a few days ago, and you told me how you felt about it. How can you now say she made it up?"

I was confronting "him" here as if "he" were now the same person I had talked to a few days earlier.

"For a while there," "he" said, "she had me believing I did it. She went out and screwed on the playground. Someone got a little rough with her. She wanted to get rid of me, so she told her mother I did it."

"What's the truth?"

"What's she been telling you is the truth? I'm telling you the truth, man."

"Which is?"

"Believe what you want . . . I sure would like to go fishing today. Do you fish?"

"I have, but I don't now."

"No, I don't really want to go fishing," "he" said.

"How about fishing into the past?"

"What do you mean?"

"I'd like to know more about your relation with Ruth."

"Look, I didn't mean to hurt her. If she'd have just not been so goddamned stubborn and not fought me. If she had just lain there, and been still, and listened to what I told her, she wouldn't have gotten hurt."

"What had you told her?"

"That I loved her, that I wanted to have her, that I'd be so good to her, that I'd make her feel good. She got that damned little snotty look on her face."

"How were you feeling?"

"Good, man. Good all over. The only trouble was I couldn't get it in. I don't know why I couldn't. She wasn't that little. I know she'd done it before."

"Oh? With whom?"

"All those little boys, probably."

"You know or you think?"

"I just know. I can tell by looking at someone. I look at her when she comes to the door, and she's so guilty-looking."

"You mean she was having intercourse at ten?"

"Screwing."

"What does that mean?"

"Intercourse."

"You think that as she was screwing, you were entitled to screw her?"

"Why not? I'm her daddy. I should be first in line . . . Do you think she would now?"

"What do you think?"

"I hope so. If she would just let me touch her one time. You know I can get a hard-on just thinking about her . . . I used to be handsome. If she'd seen me then, she'd have let me love her. I'd have always been good to her if she'd have let me. I'd have been inside of her. I got to get there."

"What would you have if you were inside her?"

I received no answer. Ruth put her face into her hands.

I asked, "Finished?"

She nodded.

"How are you feeling?"

"The same as usual. Dizzy, almost faint, shaky. Tell me how it went."

"Do you remember it?"

"No. As soon as he started to go into me, I went kind of blank."

"What do you mean, 'He started to go into me'?"

"I mean that his apparition came to me. But then I became him. The more I relaxed, the less I *saw* him and the more I *became* him."

As usual, I read my notes to her. When I'd finished, she said, "That was very tiring. It left me drained . . . I've talked about wanting to help him, but I don't think I'm the one who could do it. When you were reading the part about the rape just now, I relived it. Actually, I feel I relive it every time I look at him . . . The first thing I'm going to do when I get home is throw away that braid that's in the Bible."

The next day Ruth said, "Last night I dreamed that my father was in my bedroom. In the dream I was in the bedroom with him, standing up. I also knew I was really lying in bed, dreaming. Well, in this dream he's saying to the me that's standing up that I should stop working with you, that I should tell you I've got cold feet. Those were his words. I answer that I've got no intention of stopping. He says that I've always been wicked, but that this time it's going to hurt me. I say again that I won't stop. He says he's got no intention of leaving until I've changed my mind. That's all I remember of the dream. The me lying in bed dreaming wasn't upset, but the me standing up was angry—angry, not frightened—that he had the nerve to tell me what to do."

Her dream could mean that she was in conflict about continuing our work, perhaps because the trance experiences were making her suffer. The father of her dream could have represented her wishing to stop, and the Ruth of her dream her wishing to go on. I recognized that although she hated her father (and the "father" of the trances), she probably also felt loyal to him and perhaps guilty about exposing him to me during the trances.

Possibly she wanted to stop, but felt too desirous of pleasing me to say so.

"How do you feel about going on with the trances?" I asked.

"I don't enjoy them, and I don't like what comes out in them. But I think we should go on, because we're learning things."

"Are there any questions you'd like me to ask your father when you're in a trance?"

"Ask him about his past, his childhood, and what possessed him to feel unnatural love—and hate—for me."

"Anything else?"

"No. Just please don't make him mad when he's using my body."

"All right."

I wanted to try to find out more about who "he" really was. The actual father had never been to England. Did the person speaking to me know that "he" was in Ruth's home? The actual father had never met me or heard of me. Did "he" know who I was? Did "he" know that "he" was using Ruth's voice in talking to me? If "he" felt "his" face, would it feel beardless, as Ruth's face obviously was, or bearded? Did "he" know "he" was in possession, so to speak, of Ruth?

"I feel like a traitor," Ruth said. "Let's talk about his good characteristics. If you were hungry and barefoot in the street, he'd take you home, feed you, and give you money. He's not selfish. One reason he's not successful is he's given away so much to people. If one of my children were sick, he'd walk as far as he had to in order to get a doctor. If I were ever in trouble, he'd help me."

She paused, looked at me, and looked away. "One other thing. I'd like Paul to be here in the living room when I do it, so he doesn't feel left out. All right?"

"Yes."

We were in the living room. She went to fetch Paul from the dining room. I was curious to see whether anything unusual would happen when the three men currently in her life were in the room at the same time: her "father," Paul, and I.

She returned with Paul and asked him softly, "Do you mind if I do that thing of becoming my father in front of you?"

"No," he said. He seemed uncertain about why he was there and what might be expected of him.

She said to him, "Don't look at me as I do it. All right?"

He nodded.

She sat down on the couch, Paul sat to her right, and I sat opposite her. Again she was not going to use a mirror.

She looked at me. "I won't tell you when to start," she said. "Just start in a little while. If I'm not ready then, I'll tell you." She stared straight ahead, her eyes half-closed. She was sitting comfortably, one foot on the floor and the other foot curled under that one. One hand rested in her lap, and the other hand clutched a seat cover.

About thirty seconds passed. "Who are you?" I asked.

"Wait just another few seconds," was the reply.

I waited about a minute this time. The figure's breathing became harder, and the head and neck trembled.

"Who are you?" I asked again.

"You know who I am."

"How do you feel about being here?"

"I don't have any choice."

"Where are you?"

"In a room with you."

"Where is that room?"

"It's on a street."

"In what town?"

"I don't know."

"Are you far from home or near home?"

"I don't know."

"Do you know who I am?"

"You're Ruth's friend."

"Do you know how I got to be her friend?"

The figure laughed lewdly. "Probably."

"She came to me because you were disturbing her. You know what I mean?"

"Yeah. She doesn't want me to be near her. It's because she has no control over me."

"You recall that we've talked about the experience you and Ruth had when she was ten."

"What do you mean?"

"Oh, you know, the sexual thing."

"How do you know I did anything?"

"She told me."

"I don't want to talk to you. I don't even like you. Why should I tell you anything? I think I know what you're after. You'd like to have me locked up in jail, just so you could be with her."

Given this response, I decided not to ask about the father's childhood and his "unnatural love and hate" for Ruth, which she had wanted me to ask about.

Instead I changed the subject. "Can you tell me how your voice sounds to you?"

"Like it normally sounds. What kind of question is that?"

"I'd like to ask you something else."

"Ask me, but you don't know if I'll be lying. I think I already know what you're going to ask."

"What's that?"

"You want to know about . . . No, you don't. You thought you had me fooled."

"I want to ask you this. Could you feel your face and tell me what you feel?"

The figure placed its hands on its face and moved the fingers around on the cheeks. "What do you want to know?"

"Do you feel a beard?"

"Well, I shaved awhile ago."

"When?"

"About three hours ago."

"To return to Ruth, what's your relation with her like these days?"

"I always know her thoughts," was the answer.

"Could you give an example?"

"I don't need one."

"What do you mean when you say you always know her thoughts?"

"I don't have to answer. Man, this is getting to me."

"Do you think she knows your thoughts?"

"At times— . . . Oh, man, this trip is over."

Ruth dropped her head in her hands, took a deep breath, and lay down. "I feel dizzy," she said.

I waited a moment. "Your 'father' was more guarded and withholding than ever before in my experience," I said. "Is it possible 'he' knew Paul was here and was being more careful?"

"Maybe," she said. "He does put on an act in front of people."

Maybe it was Ruth putting on the act, restraining herself in front of Paul.

Paul, as if to ensure that no one blamed him for the unproductive session, commented to Ruth, "You—or your father—didn't once look my way."

I read my notes of the session for Ruth's benefit. I reached the part where the "father" charged me with wanting "him" locked up in jail so I could be with Ruth.

"He's always accused me of having a sexual relationship with any man I had contact with," Ruth said. "That's typical of him."

I finished reading the notes. "I don't think I heard you read one cussword in that conversation," she said. "That's unusual for him unless someone else is around. I think he'd ordinarily have told you to get the hell out of there."

I wasn't sure if the reticence of the "father" was related to Paul's presence (though the absence of cusswords probably was). Possibly Ruth had undergone a change of heart about the trances generally, despite her having said she hadn't. I thought I might find out by doing one without Paul.

The next time Ruth and I tried we were alone, sitting at her dining-room table.

She began to stare at the other side of the room. After a moment she said, "I can see his apparition perfectly, but—I hate to tell you this—I don't seem to be able to do it. I can't get rid of my own feelings."

She continued staring. Her face got tense, and her breathing became hard.

"O.K. It's beginning to happen now," she said. The next words were "his." "You don't have to speak to me. I know you're in here."

"Do you want to speak to me?" I asked.

"Yeah. Could you tell me how to do it?"

"Do what?"

"Get into her. Go on, talk about it. Tell me how to do it. If you do that, I'll tell you anything you want to know. If you don't, I'm not telling you anything. You tell me some, and I'll tell you some."

"You mean get into her sexually?"

"Yeah."

"I can't."

"Then what are you doing here? You're not so smart, are you? I'm wasting my time with you. You've got nothing to do with me. I'm none of your business. And another thing. She doesn't bring me here."

"How do you get here?"

"I stay here. Write that down . . . Do you know she's afraid of me?"

I didn't answer.

"She is. I like that. It means she knows I'm a man."

"Have you frightened any other women besides your own daughter?"

"Maybe if you begged me, I might tell you. 'Would you please tell me?' Shit, I've got no time to fool with you."

Ruth laid her head on the table. She was perspiring visibly and breathing very deeply. "I feel tired, and shaky, and cold," she said. "I think this time we overdid it." Her hands were trembling. "Did anything strenuous happen? I feel as if it did."

"Your body didn't move at all, if that's what you mean by 'strenuous.' What do you remember?"

"Only that it was hard to begin with . . . Even my chin was shaking." The whole upper part of her body was now trembling.

"I know there must be something that happened in that session or I wouldn't be trembling this way. I've got to get up."

She walked around the room for about three minutes, trying to calm down, but still trembling.

When she had relaxed, I read back the session to her.

"I'm feeling numb," she commented. "He certainly seemed smug. What I dislike most is his saying that I'm afraid of him."

I tried to understand what had been happening in these sessions. Perhaps she had been consciously enacting a role that portrayed her actual father's personality. If so, it was an extraordinary performance.

Why had she remembered so little of the sessions afterward? Maybe this was a way of dramatizing her apparent transformation into another person; she would have no memory of the experiences if they were genuinely her father's.

However, I wondered whether she would really have gone to such lengths to enact a performance for me. I looked for other possible interpretations of her trances. I recalled a most peculiar phenomenon that has been observed for centuries, in which a person seems to be taken over by another person or by a "spirit" or "demon." The phenomenon has attracted much interest but still has not received full interpretation. It manifests in various ways depending on the culture. People give up their ordinary style of dressing, talking, eating, and thinking, without apparently wanting to. It is as if they become vehicles for the expression of beings other than themselves, whose manner and character differ from their own. One's original personality can be replaced for a moment, or for days, weeks, or even years. If a person is taken over by one alien personality, it is called a case of dual personality; if there is more than one alien personality, each one assuming charge for some time, it is called a case of multiple personality.

While one personality, especially the original personality, is in command, it is often ignorant of any of the other personalities' experiences. Similarly, Ruth had recalled little or nothing about what happened while her "father" was in charge. In this regard she had resembled a trance medium, who does not usually remember what has occurred while under the control of another personality.

In the childhoods of dual and multiple personality cases, brutality, sadism, and sexual assaults have commonly occurred, as they did in Ruth's childhood.

In dual or multiple personality, shifts from one personality to another are generally outside any personality's voluntary control. Ruth had deliberately substituted another personality for her own, as trance mediums do.

What was I to make of the "father" of her trances? The fact of "his" speaking through her at all was startling, to say the least. Though she did not know what questions I would ask "him" or how I would word them, "he" was able to answer them spontaneously and convincingly. Not having met the father, I could not tell how closely he resembles the character she portrayed. Nor could I say whether "he" was giving information about her father's actual past or feelings that was otherwise unavailable to her. The "father" gave a remarkably plausible psychological picture of a person who might have treated Ruth as her actual father had allegedly done. Much of what "he" said was consistent with the person she had described her father to be and was uncharacteristic of the Ruth I knew.

However, there were reasons for regarding the personality in the room with me in these trances as being Ruth herself. Firstly, the personality seemed for the most part to talk comfortably with me and to see me as someone familiar. As the actual father did not know me, he could not have done so. Secondly, although the personality apparently experienced the father's emotions, these emotions were not displayed, and no action based upon them was taken; the figure remained seated and virtually motionless throughout the trances. Since Ruth had described the actual father to me as impulsive in his actions, this behavior did not coincide with that description.

I thought she was representing in the trances either her actual father (except in the two respects mentioned) or a buried aspect of herself.[17] These two types of interpretation do not exclude one another and are probably both true.

One way that people, especially children, deal with threats from others is to identify with the persons threatening them. After receiving an injection from a doctor, a child sometimes plays at injecting a doll or a younger sibling. Mimicking an attacker's behavior represents a primitive way of trying to master the attack. But the identification cannot simply be understood as imitative behavior. It is the self's attempt to relinquish its view of itself as a victim, by means of merging its identity with the aggressor's.

As a child, Ruth may have tried to cope with her feelings about her father's sexual assault upon her by uniting with him. She had once said:

. . . There's a strong feeling between him and me. In a way I'm closer to him than to anyone else in the world. I find it hard to explain the feeling. It's not a closeness in the sense that we confide in each other. It's that there's so much going on emotionally between us.

What I am suggesting accords with Ruth's remarks made in a dream about the apparition of herself:

Dr. Schatzman, I know she is angry, very angry, and I don't dare let that anger out of her. I'm afraid she'll behave like my daddy did. The anger is like a great ball of fire. If it starts to roll, I don't think I'll be able to stop it. I'm really talking about myself, you know.

If Ruth had identified as a child with her father, she had incorporated representations of him into herself.[18] That was who the "father" of her trances might be. If her father is embedded in some sense within her, the sexual excitement that wet her panties during the trances could be seen as either his or hers. Wherever he is within her, distinctions between her feelings and his are blurred.

In one of the trance sessions, the "father" said:

> I've got to do it, be inside her, to be inside each drop of blood . . . I want to be all inside, to crawl up inside of her.

> If I get in, I'll stay and never come back out.

> I'd have her all around me . . . I want to be in her and in the blood. I want to be deep in her, as deep as deep can be. I want her to close up all around me.

Perhaps Ruth's actual father had really wanted what the "father" of this trance session wanted. Perhaps that is why he tried to rape her. And perhaps Ruth unconsciously recognized his want, and granted it—psychologically, not sexually.

What I have been saying can explain the phenomena of Ruth's trances only partially—many people presumably identify with aggressors and yet cannot do what she did in these trances. The full interpretation of her trance behavior may need to await further understanding of trance mediumship and cases of multiple personality.

And now, it is time to resume Ruth's story.

Sorrow and Play

R UTH had gone to America for her grandmother's funeral, taking her children with her, but Paul had had to stay in England.

A little over a week after Ruth left, Paul sent on to me a letter from her.

Dear Morty,

. . . I went to the funeral home with knots in my stomach. I couldn't swallow. The smell of the flowers there frightened me. I walked into a crowded room, where everybody called me Cheepy. I could tell I looked bad, because they wanted to console me. I hated all of them who hadn't been close to her. I walked into another room where the coffin was. I couldn't believe she was dead. She looked so real, only younger. She had on a blue satin gown with long sleeves and a high collar laced around the neck. She looked beautiful. She was cold, and her flesh felt hard. I couldn't stand up any longer. I sat in a chair near her. They were going to bury her in two hours. I stayed by her until they moved her to the chapel. I felt closer to her than I had in my whole life. Everyone kept telling my mama that I needed her, but I didn't. I wanted to cry and mourn all alone. At the chapel service I couldn't stand it. The preacher meant well, but he kept saying things he knew nothing about. They played her favorite hymns, which she used to sing to me when she rocked me. I didn't break down, because Grandma had said never to show your feelings for outsiders to see. Then we drove to the cemetery and had another service. They put her in a hole and piled dirt on her. It was awful. I don't remember anything after that for a while.

Not that night but the next one, I dreamed that Grandma was standing in that dress at my bedroom door. Her arms were outstretched, and she told me to come with her. She said I wouldn't have to go alone if I'd come now. I told her I was afraid to go with her. She said for me to please hurry, because she had to go right then. She was backing out of the door begging me. I knew it was a dream and I was afraid. . . .

I'm afraid of having apparitions of her. I don't know why. I haven't been able to do any apparitions of my father. I'm too upset about Grandma and too afraid of him.

Ruth

About ten days later her next letter to me came.

Dear Morty,

. . . I understand so much more about my Daddy and I'm beginning to see him as a different person. He still has some sort of deep dislike of me. I don't think he realizes it. He's more fatherly toward me than he's ever been. We talk and seem to enjoy each other's company. . . .

. . . I've been playing with my ability. Mallory and her husband have a restaurant near our home. Occasionally in the evenings I've been helping out there as a waitress. As I watch customers come in, I make apparitions of them standing at the cash register ready to leave. I hallucinate the bill the cashier gives them. Later, when they've really finished, I see what bill gets flashed upon the cash register. Well—a mind reader I'm not. Not one apparition has paid the same amount as the real customer. One woman amazed me. She came in, and I hallucinated her paying $18.22. I never thought she'd reach that amount, but she did. Her bill was $18.22. . . .

Love,

Ruth

Ruth wasn't really trying to mind-read; she was trying to predict the future. There was no reason to expect her to have a skill at prediction just because she could produce apparitions. But I thought it might be useful to test whether she could procure information from an apparition where the information was known to the person whose apparition it was, but not to her.

She was away for four weeks. The day after she returned, I went to visit her at home. She was pleased to see me, but seemed somehow restrained.

Paul and the children were there. He and Ruth had introduced me as their friend to the children, since Ruth did not want them to know that I had been her therapist or that we were working with apparitions.

"She's already filled me in on things," Paul said to me. "I guess she's got a lot to tell you." He put some logs on the fire in the living room where we were sitting, brought us some coffee, and then went out with the dog and the children.

"My father's much older than I remember," she began. "His

health is broken. He says he's dying, but I don't know of what.
"He treated me better than before. He showed me respect. I'd
ask him a question about something in his past, and he'd go on and
on about it, telling me things. He used to say, 'It's none of your
damned business,' or 'Why are you so concerned about me?'
"He told me some of his dreams too. They've all got killing and
bleeding in them. He never seems to be inflicting violence. He's
the victim of it or just watching it.
"Wherever he goes he takes his guns. He always keeps a loaded,
high-powered rifle with him. He doesn't offer any explanations—
he doesn't feel he owes any."
I commented, "Maybe he's trying to protect himself from the
violence of his dreams."
She made no reply.
"He's still up to an old trick of his," she said, "walking in on me
while I'm dressing. He did it a few times. I'd say, 'Daddy, I'm
dressing.' He'd say, 'Oh, yeah,' and walk out."
Since this had occurred more than once, I wondered if she had
been inviting him in, half-deliberately—or at least had not been
taking care to keep him out. I did not say so, since I wanted to
hear what else she had to say.
"One sunny morning I was downtown shopping with him and
my children. In one shop the children were so excited by the toys
on the counter they couldn't keep their hands off them. I was
afraid they'd break something, so I decided we'd leave. My father
left the shop with us. As we were walking out the door, I got a
brainstorm. My car was down the street, maybe twenty yards
away, and was half in shadow from a nearby tree. I made an
apparition of Paul sitting behind the steering wheel. He had
shadows across his face, but I could see him plainly. I told Daddy,
who was standing next to me, to look in the car, because I thought
someone was sitting there.
"'Oh, yeah,' he said. 'It looks like a ghost sitting in there. Isn't
that the damndest thing? It looks like a man, just like Paul!'
"My mouth dropped open. He might as well have said, 'The
leaves are dropping off the trees'—it was no big deal to him.

"I asked him if he'd ever seen anything like that before. He said, 'I could tell you things to make your hair stand up, but you'd think I was insane.'"

My mouth was sagging a bit, too. "Did he tell you any of those stories?" I asked.

"He told me that once when he'd been put in jail, a man had visited his cell and said he'd put up bail for him and get him out of there in a few hours. When visiting time was over, the jailer came and let the man out. My father kept waiting. No word came about the bail. My father asked about the man, but they didn't know what he was talking about. So, he sees apparitions too."

How had he identified Paul's apparition sitting in the car? Possibly he had made a lucky guess. Possibly Paul had driven that car, and the father, remembering him sitting behind the wheel, had imagined—or hallucinated—him there now. Possibly there was some other simple, nonparanormal explanation for what had happened. But possibly an apparition of Paul had truly been sitting in the car, visible to anyone with the power to see it. Yet how could anyone besides Ruth see an entity that she had visualized on a whim and that was presumably immaterial?

Was it possible, I wondered, for someone with a history of seeing apparitions to see the same apparitions Ruth did? I started thinking of people I knew with whom to test this, and how I might go about it.

"Perhaps your ability to experience apparitions is hereditary," I said, "in which case your children might have it too."

"I'm a step ahead of you," she replied in a tone of mock superiority. "After that thing happened with my father, I made an apparition beside the children or in front of them many times. If they had seen it, they would have had to walk around it. But they never seemed to notice a thing."

"You never made an apparition next to your father or in front of him?"

"No. I was afraid he'd see it and know I'd put it there. He's wise, and I didn't want him to get wise to me."

I thought it was a pity that she had not tested him again.

"I tried a few times to become my father," she said, "but I couldn't. When I tried, I felt strange, but I couldn't feel his feelings.

"I did have conversations with your apparition and with Paul's. In one conversation you told me that one of your children wasn't feeling well and that you were worried."

I reflected on the past few weeks. Neither of my children had been ill, and I told her so.

"Oh, I just remembered something else," she said. "I was driving with my children down a long road. It was around noon, the sun was high in the sky, and it was bright and hot—about ninety degrees. Wind was blowing dirt everywhere. We were coming back from visiting Paul's parents, where we'd spent a few days. I'd been driving for four hours and had about five hours to go. I was very tired. The road was flat. No buildings were in sight, not even farmhouses or filling stations. It was the middle of nowhere.

"I saw a black man walking along the roadside in the same direction I was driving. He was wearing a black tuxedo with tails and a top hat. His right hand was up in the air, and I could see his white cuff. He didn't seem to be going anywhere or to have come from anywhere. I wondered what he was doing there. He should have been dirty and dusty from walking on the road, but he wasn't. He looked very neat, as if he'd just stepped out of a wedding or an opera. He didn't look uncomfortable in the heat, which he should have, especially the way he was dressed. After passing him, I looked in the rearview mirror and saw his reflection.

"This can't be, I thought. There's nobody there. It must be an apparition. I thought that, because of his clothes and how clean and neat he was. When I looked again, he was gone. That proved it was an apparition; there was nowhere he could have disappeared to.

"The two older children were awake and were looking out the window. I'm pretty sure they didn't see anyone there, because they'd have said something.

"If I'd realized it was an apparition before passing it, I'd have stopped to look closely. I'd have wanted to see if I'd met him in the flesh before.

"Afterward I thought it could have been dangerous. I had no control over him. If he'd stepped out in front of me, I'd have swerved, and could've had an accident.

"When I told the story to Paul, he said he's been worrying too, about my driving, with all this apparitions business.

"He said, 'Now, what if it had run in front of you and you'd guessed it was an apparition and you'd run it over, and then it had turned out it wasn't?'

"That possibility bothers me. I think I've been driving more cautiously than I used to."

"I hope so," I said. "I wouldn't like you running someone over and then bringing me to court to testify, 'Yes, Your Honor, I believe she thought it was an apparition, because she's been seeing people who aren't there for a long time.'"

We both laughed.

"When I walk down the street now," she said, "I wonder how many people are real and how many are apparitions."

She got up, went out of the room, and returned a moment later. "I wanted to make sure Paul's not here before telling you this," she said. "One night I was lying in bed feeling lonely. I started making an apparition of Paul. When it appeared, it was nude and looked just like him. Neither of us said anything. I was lying on one side of the bed, and he lay down on the other beside me. He kissed me, which felt pleasant. I shut my eyes and let him kiss me more. I could feel his tongue and saliva. I could smell him too.

"He cupped a breast with one hand, and put his other hand under my back. He kissed my breasts and stomach. I could feel an urgency in him, just as if he were real. He kissed my mouth again. Then he began to make love to me. I had my arms around him and could feel his back. At first we made love slowly, then faster and faster. I was so excited I forgot it wasn't real. He was excited too. I could hear his breathing. We climaxed together. As he came, I felt his penis contract inside me, and heard him moan.

"I'd felt uncomfortable with the idea of making love to his apparition, and curious to see if I could. I did it because I was lonely.

"I did it a second time," she said.

"Oh, what happened then?"

"It was just as nice. After coming home from the restaurant, I was alone in my bedroom. This time he appeared in his shorts. He sat on the bed and took them off. He kissed me and fondled my body—not for long, not for as long as usual. Then he gently spread my legs. He made love to me pretty much the way he had before."

"How did you make him appear naked or in his shorts, ready to make love?"

"I don't know. I don't know how I make him appear with clothes on. I just thought of making love with him. When he appeared, I knew that was what he was there for."

"Did you fondle his penis?"

"No, I didn't have to. Both times he had an erection. That's usual."

"When did the apparition disappear?"

"After he'd climaxed, he was lying on top of me relaxing. That's when I made him disappear."

"Could you have had him fall asleep next to you?"

"I couldn't have fallen asleep with an apparition lying there. I'd have been too busy checking to see if it was still there."

"How satisfying was it sexually?"

"Very. If I'm ever on my own, it'll be a good substitute for Paul himself."

I said nothing.

"I wondered afterward if I'd tell you. I didn't feel guilty until I got back here and told Paul. He stared blankly. I wish he'd either approve or disapprove."

"He probably doesn't know what to feel."

"Well, he got enjoyment out of it." She laughed.

"Try and convince him of that!"

I found these experiences of Ruth, like many of her others,

extraordinary and amazing. Several hundred years ago in Europe, women commonly reported having sexual relations with a demon in their sleep or while lying awake in bed; and women were sometimes accused of such experiences, and denied them. The sort of demon who supposedly had sexual relations with a woman in bed at night was called an incubus.[19] According to tradition, an incubus could masquerade as a real person, even as the woman's own husband. Did the women realize from the start, as Ruth did, that their relations were not with a real person, or did they recognize the truth only afterward? It is difficult to tell from available information. Did the women stimulate their own genitals during their experiences? Did they reach orgasm? It is not known. At that time there was no scientific inquiry into such experiences.

Nowadays it is thought rare for a woman to reach orgasm on her own, while awake, without her stimulating her genital area rhythmically by touching it with her hand or an instrument, by moving it against a soft object, or by pressing her thighs together. The two American sex-researchers, William H. Masters and Virginia E. Johnson, who observed in a laboratory more than 7500 orgasms in 382 women, found no woman who could fantasize to orgasm—that is, who could reach orgasm without receiving genital stimulation.[20] It is possible that their research subjects found the laboratory situation inhibiting.

"While Paul's apparition was making love to you," I asked Ruth, "did you touch your genitals with your finger?"

"No, I'm sure I didn't. My arms were around Paul."

"Were your thighs or pelvis moving up and down?"

"I was too busy enjoying myself to think about it."

Even if she had felt herself moving up and down, she might not have actually been moving, since she had felt an apparition raise her leg, when her leg had not actually moved.

I saw these sexual experiences as representing a special personal triumph for Ruth. From the start of her recent crisis, an apparition had been interfering in her sexual life with Paul. As a result, she and Paul had doubted whether their marriage could survive. By exploiting the potential of an apparition's sexual presence, she had now transformed adversity into advantage. Formerly, against her will, she had seen Paul change into her father's apparition during lovemaking. Now, she had willed Paul's apparition into existence to make love to it. Whereas the former experience had terrified her, the latter ones had delighted her.

We heard the front door open. Paul was back with the children and the dog.

We all had lunch together.

After lunch, the children went into the living room, and Ruth followed them to play with them. Paul and I remained sitting at the dining-room table.

"What did you feel," I asked him, "about Ruth visiting her family and being around her father again?"

"Worry. Fear that if she went back her whole emotional thing might start again."

"What about the possibility of violence to her by her father?"

"With someone like him, there's always a risk. It was in the back of my mind. But she'd decided to go, and I wasn't free to go with her."

He looked down at the table for a long moment and cleared his throat. "The company I've been working for," he said, "is nearing completion of the contract I've been working on in England. I'd known about that for a few months. But until a few days ago, I'd thought there was a good chance of another contract. That's fallen through, which means we'll be returning to the United States in a few weeks."

"Does Ruth know yet?"

"I told her last night."

That might account, I thought, for my feeling that her greeting to me had been restrained.

"Will she be all right?" he asked. "Do you think her problems could return?"

I was asking myself the same questions.

"She's gone through a lot and come out of it well," I said. "I'm pretty sure she'll be O.K., but I can't be certain. If anything comes up, phone me, and I'll do all I can to help."

While Ruth and Paul were still in England, they played a game which she told me about. The game was Paul's idea.

His plan was to go out and buy some pairs of underpants. When he got back he would put on a pair out of sight of Ruth, dress again, and enter the living room where she was. She would then make an apparition of him, naked except for the underpants, and describe the underpants the apparition was wearing.

She agreed to try.

Paul changed into the new underpants and returned to the living room.

"All right," Ruth said, "your apparition is here and is dressed. Now he's unbuckling his trousers and unzipping them. He's pulling them down. He's got on some black nylon or satin bikini briefs. Something is written on the front of them. There's a clock face with the little hand on the six and the big hand on the twelve, and underneath are the words 'early riser.'"

Paul laughed. "Where did you ever see underpants like those?"

"Probably in a shop. Can I see if I'm right?" Paul took off his trousers. He was wearing tight-fitting yellow nylon shorts with brown borders and no writing on them. They were not bikini pants.

"I'm disappointed," Ruth told me. "But I don't think I'm a mind reader."

"The outcome of that game doesn't surprise me," I said. "You, not Paul, chose the underpants of Paul's apparition, just as you, not the people the apparitions represent, have generally controlled the apparitions."

"Why do you say *generally* controlled, instead of *always?*"

"Because of the possibility that your grandmother had something to do with her apparition manifesting on the day she died—though I doubt she did."

I remembered Ruth saying that the apparitions had personalities and that she couldn't make them act as she wanted them to.

I wondered if Paul's apparition had chosen on a whim to wear its own underpants and not to copy Paul. But should I entertain the possibility that an apparition was a separate being with its own consciousness and will? That was what her father's apparition had alleged in the midst of her crisis. I had repeatedly told her, and believed, that her father's apparition was a product of her own mind and had no independent existence. However, I was still also considering a more improbable, more audacious possibility, without actually believing it.

I went on musing to myself. "If the apparitions are actually capable of willfulness, and if they wish to interfere with our experiments into the paranormal, our experiments will be affected."

A whimsical voice within me whispered, "Perhaps an apparition of you will be more cooperative than Paul's was. Your desire for Ruth's success might be stronger than Paul's, as you have a professional interest in her success."

"But," I answered, "an apparition of me is a creation of Ruth's mind, not mine. It couldn't be an agent of my wishes."

"Couldn't it?" was the whimsical voice's faint reply.

My speculations continued. "If Ruth tried to obtain from my apparition information known to me that she ordinarily had no access to, would her success depend upon my transmitting the information paranormally, upon her eliciting it, or upon both? And what if my apparition had a will of its own, subject neither to my wishes nor to hers?" But I did not give that possibility much weight.

I enjoyed playing with these outlandish thoughts. However, I recognized that these thoughts were unsupported by positive experimental results. It was time to do some tests.

"Why don't you produce an apparition of me and see if you can find out some things about me?" I said to Ruth one day in my office.

"Such as?"

"Whatever you like."

"Anything?"

I laughed. "Anything about some things. Anyway, it's between you and my apparition. I can't stop you if you want to pry."

"The idea of that sort of power scares me, but it also tempts me. I'll try. How about if I ask the apparition for details of your children's births?"

"Fine."

Ruth already knew that I had two sons, Daniel and Gideon, and their ages, and that my wife's name was Vivien.

She said, "I'm making the apparition now . . . It's here . . . I'm asking it where Daniel was born . . . He was born in a hospital."

"That's right. What's the name of the hospital?"

"St. James."

"In fact, it's called University College Hospital."

"Gideon was born at home."

"Right."

I thought that since many women in England deliver their first babies in a hospital and their second ones at home—which Ruth, who had been living in England, could have known—her performance was unremarkable, though encouraging.

"An image just came to me," Ruth said, "of a room in which your wife is giving birth. I'm imagining the scene, not actually seeing it. A gray-haired woman is there. She's grumpy. I feel Vivien doesn't like her."

"There was a woman like that there, a gray-haired, grumpy midwife. I don't think though that Vivien disliked her. Do you see me in that room?"

"No."

"In fact, I was in the room when Gideon was born. Let's try another topic."

"All right."

"Soon after finishing my formal psychiatric training, I lived for a year in a community with people whom most psychiatrists would consider schizophrenic. Why don't you ask my apparition about that community?"

She asked the apparition about the building the community had lived in, the street the building was on, the people composing the community, and so on.

The apparition scored some hits, but they were unimpressive, and its misses far outnumbered the hits.

On another occasion, she asked my apparition about my present-day friends: their names, other identifying features, things they and I had done together, and so on.

Again the hits were few and unimpressive.

I persisted with this line of research, despite the results so far, because I knew that if Ruth could somehow find a way of achieving hits regularly, this would be most interesting and important.

Ruth produced an apparition of me in my office to ask it questions about mental illness. Obviously I had knowledge about mental illness that she lacked. The question remained the same: could the apparition know something that Ruth did not know?

She asked the apparition to say something about the different kinds of schizophrenia.

She said to me, "He's saying, 'There are different types. There's paranoid schizophrenia.'

"I've heard of that before," she commented.

"He's explaining, 'A person becomes angry and violent if he feels other people are laughing at him, mocking him, or even looking at him. Such a person could be set off and assault someone.'"

This statement accurately describes some people who are considered paranoid schizophrenics. However, since it also describes Ruth's father, whom she believed had been labeled schizophrenic, she already had this information.

The apparition did not mention any other kind of schizophrenia.

The apparition said that suicidal feelings are a cry for help, and that Ruth had not really wanted to die, but that she would have killed herself had she not received help. Ruth told the apparition she would not have killed herself. The apparition said that she was wrong and that it was right.

I did not favor either opinion, though I found it interesting that Ruth and the apparition could disagree. Perhaps Ruth was practicing becoming independent of me by disagreeing with my apparition and by telling it she would have survived without my help.

Could an apparition convey to Ruth information about objects that were out of her line of vision?

I held in my hands some postcard-size reproductions of paintings. From where she was sitting, she could see only the backs of the cards. I asked her to create an apparition standing behind me so that it could see the fronts of the cards and try to make it tell her what was on the cards.

She used an apparition of me.

We tried with three cards, one at a time. Each time the apparition reported seeing something on the card, but its reports did not resemble what was on the cards.

Another time I positioned a clock with its face to me and its back to Ruth. She made an apparition of me facing the clock. At first, the apparition refused to tell her the time; later, when it did, it told her that the clock read 3:20. In fact, the clock showed the time to be 11:45.

All these experiments using the apparition of me had yielded the same results: Ruth had acquired no correct information from the apparition that she had not already had access to. This did not necessarily mean that such a feat was beyond her. Perhaps she might have succeeded with practice, or under different conditions. Meanwhile, the evidence from the paintings and clock experiments suggested that the apparitions were unable to obtain information that she did not have, and I pointed this out to her. Given the limited amount of time available to us, I decided we ought to spend it on other sorts of research.

Even before Ruth had told me of her father seeing Paul's

apparition, I had heard of apparitions being experienced by more than one person at once.[21] I wondered if I could encourage the phenomenon to occur in my presence. Ruth's father was unavailable for research, but perhaps someone else could see an apparition produced by her. If someone could I would consider it very remarkable.

Ruth decided to try again to test whether her children, George, aged seven, and Heather, now aged four, could see an apparition. This time I wanted to watch the experiment myself.

As far as Ruth was aware, the children did not know of her ability to produce apparitions—and she did not want them to know.

Her idea was to play "I Spy" with them, a game which is played like this. One person says, "I spy blue (or red, or any color), and it's by that wall (or on the floor, or on a table, or somewhere else)." The other persons must then say what the first person has spied.

Ruth whispered in my ear that she was going to produce an apparition of Becky wearing a blue blouse and blue jeans and standing against a wall in the living room.

Ruth pointed to the wall. "I spy blue and it's by that wall," she said.

"I see it," Heather said.

"Yes?" said Ruth.

"It's a blue button on the tape recorder."

"Anyone see anything else blue?"

George and Heather were silent.

Ruth whispered again in my ear. "I guess they can't see it, but maybe they can hear it."

She turned to them. "Someone—it might be me, or Morty, or someone else—is going to whisper something. When someone does, I want whoever hears it to tell me what they hear. All right?"

George and Heather nodded.

Ruth said, "I hear with my little ears something being whispered . . . NOW."

George and Heather said nothing.

"I hear with my little ears something being whispered . . . NOW."

Again they said nothing.

"I hear with my little ears something being whispered . . . NOW."

Heather said, "I hear a duck quacking."

George asked, "Did someone whisper, 'Go wash your hands for supper'?"

Ruth turned to me and said softly, "I'd had Becky say three times, 'Heather, do you hear me?'"

We played similar games with my own two children, who are close in age to George and Heather. We concealed the real purpose of the games from my children too. They did not see or hear the apparitions either.

I knew three adults who had experienced a visual hallucination more than once while fully awake and who did not suffer from a mental disorder. All agreed to try, as research subjects, to see an apparition produced by Ruth.

One of the research subjects, Ruth, and I sat facing a wall in a room with partitions between us, so that we could each see the whole wall, but not each other. I sat in the middle, with the research subject on my left and Ruth on my right. To prevent the subject from hearing any sounds Ruth might make, he wore earphones that transmitted continuous low-volume noise from a machine.

Before the subject had entered the room, I had shuffled eighteen envelopes and handed six of them to Ruth, who was already sitting in her chair; then I had sat in mine. Each envelope contained a file card on which Ruth had described in detail an apparition.

Ruth now opened an envelope, read the file card, and started to produce by the wall facing her the apparition described on the card. As she did, she turned a knob next to her. The knob was connected to a lamp that was visible to the research subject, and Ruth could control the intensity of its light with the knob. That way she could inform the subject when an apparition was coming into being, how vivid it was, and when it was disappearing.

The subject had to mark on a checklist where the apparition was, whether it was standing, sitting, crouching, or kneeling; its age; its hair color; its hair length; if its hair was wavy, straight, or curly; if it was bald, partly bald, or had a full head of hair; if it was bearded; if it was heavy, medium, or light in weight; its approximate height; the color of whatever it was wearing above the waist; and the color of whatever it was wearing below the waist. The subject was asked to describe the apparition's mood and its feelings toward people in the room. After finishing each checklist, the subject pressed a buzzer to tell Ruth it was time for the next apparition.

Each of the three subjects received six chances to see an apparition. Ruth said that all eighteen times she managed to produce the apparition described on the file card, though some were only faint and fleeting. After each apparition had faded away, she wrote down any further observations she had made about it.

All three subjects occasionally sensed and even glimpsed figures against the wall coinciding in time with Ruth's production of apparitions. However—and this is the crucial point—the characteristics of those figures and of the apparitions that Ruth was creating at the same time did not correspond even once.

The result meant that under these conditions Ruth had been unable to transmit—or the subjects had been unable to detect—images of the apparitions.

Ruth left England six weeks after having returned from her grandmother's funeral. When she left, I thought it might be the end of our collaborative work. However, this was not so. A year later, at my request, she arranged to come back without her family to do two more weeks of research.

Three weeks before she was due to arrive again in England, my phone rang at 5:00 A.M., London time.

"Hello?" I said.

"Hi!" It was Ruth. "Sorry to be phoning you at this hour. I know I'm waking you. But I felt if I didn't phone, I'd explode."

"Yes?" It occurred to me that she had never phoned me transatlantic before.

"Paul was sitting in the kitchen. He said, 'On your trip to England, if you visit the village we used to live in, could you go up to the pub and have a drink there for me? And could you say hello to our friends?'

"I laughed and said, 'I might meet some good-looking guy there.'

"'No, you don't,' he said, and he laughed. Then he stood up and walked over to the wastepaper basket to empty it into the garbage can outside. As he was picking up the basket, he looked at me. When he saw me sitting in the chair near the front door, where I'd been sitting all along, he stopped as if he'd seen a ghost. He said, 'You were just sitting on the sofa. How did you get over to that chair?' The sofa was several yards from where I'd been sitting.

"I asked Paul, 'In what position had I been sitting on the sofa?'

"He said, 'She sat on the sofa and pulled her feet under her so that she was sitting on her feet.'

"I said, 'That was an apparition of me you saw on the sofa! Before you started to talk to me, I'd made the apparition and had been talking to it in my mind about whether the plane I'd be on to England would crash. It was still there while you and I were talking. I've been sitting in my chair the whole time and haven't moved from it. I haven't been near the sofa.'

"Paul nearly went up the wall. He said, 'I'm catching this business of seeing apparitions from you. It's rubbing off on me.'

"I told him, 'That can't be.'

"He wasn't at all reassured. He said, 'I feel as if I'm going crazy. Laura and Andrea better keep a room open for me at the Crisis Centre.'

"Now, what do you think of that?" Ruth said to me.

"I think it's a remarkable event."

Three weeks later, in my office, Ruth told me more about it.

"Until Paul went for the trash," she explained, "he hadn't looked in the direction of the real me."

"From where had he heard your voice coming?" I asked.

"I asked him the same question. He'd heard my voice coming from the sofa, where the apparition was. He'd also seen the apparition's mouth moving as if it had been saying the words that I'd actually been saying."

"I'm puzzled about how the apparition's mouth came to be moving," I said. "You weren't directing the apparition at the time, as your thoughts had turned to the conversation with Paul. Perhaps he put the mouth movements there."

"Yes, perhaps."

"Did he tell you what the apparition was wearing?"

"Yes. The same things I was wearing: panties and a T-shirt that said Donald Duck across the chest. I'd gotten it as a memento from Disneyland. That's how I'd seen the apparition dressed."

"How much light was in the room?"

"Outside it was dark. In the room was a ceiling light, which wasn't very bright."

"What happened to the apparition when Paul realized that that was what he'd been seeing?" I asked.

"When he saw the real me in my chair, he looked at the sofa, and then back at me. I stopped making the apparition.

"He was very upset about what had happened. In bed that night he felt me all over, saying, 'Is that you?' I teased him. I said, 'You can't be sure.' He made me promise on our marriage vow I'd never again do an apparition in a room with him. At three A.M. he woke me up to get me to promise again. I think he's been suspecting me since then of playing tricks on him by having an apparition of me talk to him in one room, while I'm really in another room. But he's wrong.

"Do you think Paul could have seen the apparition because he was run-down and tired?" she asked.

"It may have contributed, but I don't think it's enough of an explanation in itself. How do you know that the person you thought was Paul wasn't an apparition?" I asked with a smile.

"Because he lasted too long," she answered. "The apparitions never last more than a few minutes, but Paul stayed there for the whole evening."

I phoned Paul and asked him about the event in detail. "Yes, it happened just as she told it to you," he said. "I can't explain it. I wish someone could."

Was there a satisfactory explanation? I considered several possibilities, but felt content with none of them.

I now threw into question a basic conclusion that the apparitions produced by Ruth were only her private experiences. If Paul had seen Ruth's apparition and if the father had seen Paul's apparition, it meant that someone besides Ruth could see the apparitions. Yet the range-finder experiment had established that the apparitions were not sending out ordinary light rays the way an actual person does. And we had been unable to photograph an apparition. So I did not understand how it was possible for someone else to have seen one. Nor did I understand how an apparition could have been visible once to the father and once to Paul, but not to anyone on any other occasion. If there was someone available who could repeatedly experience the apparitions Ruth created, I could explore these matters.

"My father hasn't changed his ways," Ruth said. "After leaving England, I visited my parents with Paul and the children. My father took hold of my son George and held a gun to his head. My father said, 'I'm going to do it. I'm going to do it.' A neighbor grabbed my father from behind, talked him out of it, and took the gun away from him.

"I wonder if my father will ever change. I know I'll keep my distance from him.

"During the past year, I've had some beautiful experiences with my grandmother. I've remembered, imagined, and seen her. She seems to know the things I need to hear, because she tells them to me before I even try to ask. And she explains them so beautifully.

"One evening I was awake in bed. I'd been wondering if death was dark. Grandma appeared, looking real. She said she was never afraid, and I shouldn't be. I asked her if she was waiting for Jesus or a Messiah to come. She said she wasn't waiting for anyone. I asked her if she was where she was always going to be. She said she was where she'd always been, and she smiled in a way that said she knew I didn't understand what she was talking about, but someday I would.

"I told her I felt her presence constantly, and I asked her if she was really there. Her answer was yes. I asked her if reincarnation was what kept life going on. She told me not to try to get her to answer that. I asked her if I could touch her, and she said I couldn't.

"I asked if she knew about the results of the research we'd been doing. She said she knew what was in me.

"Although she looks real and not ghostlike, she's definitely different from apparitions of living people. She's more aware and has more feeling. I look upon her as my real grandmother, not as a figment of my imagination.

"She's not bathed in light and has no halo around her head. There's no rainbow or streaks of white light from heaven, and she doesn't have wings. She also doesn't look as if she's doing any time in hell.

"As an apparition, she has always looked the age she seemed to be in her coffin—in her sixties, though she was actually in her nineties—and she'd had on the same dress she had on in the coffin.

"I've noticed I can never see her feet. The room takes on a dark haze below the bottom of her dress. And as she backs off, she gets darker.

"I think the sounds I hear when she speaks are in my head, not outside, as they often seem to be when apparitions speak.

"I can't control her coming and going. Even if I could make her appear, I wouldn't feel right doing it. I don't know how people spend time when they're dead and I don't feel allowed to make them come to me. I'd rather not disturb her. I believe she comes and talks with me in my dreams or when I'm awake if she wants to and if she can, without my summoning her. Yet I'm always glad that she comes.

"Since having these experiences, I don't fear death anymore."

Memory Trances

THE unexpected from Ruth was nothing new to me, but the events I shall now relate caught me completely unawares and led us onto a fresh path altogether.

Ruth had once said that now that she could summon an apparition of herself she would never have trouble remembering anything about herself. On that occasion the apparition had told her, "Get to know yourself. Ask me questions."

I wondered what all this meant. Ruth and I decided to explore the matter. Since the "father" had been so helpful in adding to our understanding, perhaps the apparition of herself would be.

A few weeks before Ruth left England to go back to the United States, she and I were sitting in her living room.

"Shall we try to find out something about you from your apparition?" I said. "Would you be willing to summon her?"

"Yes." Ruth stared straight ahead. "All right . . . It's coming. I see her now."

"Would you ask her why you started seeing apparitions in the summer of 1976?" I had been asking myself this question.

For a few seconds Ruth stared. "She says, 'You didn't start seeing them in the summer of 1976. You played with them as a child.'"

It was an answer, but not what I had anticipated. I wanted to know why her father's apparition had begun to harass her. I knew she had experienced apparitions as a child. However, I had not heard of her playing with them and I wondered if it was true.

Ruth glanced at me. "I don't remember playing with apparitions. All my friends were real—I think. I'll ask her why I don't remember."

Ruth stared in the same direction as before. "She says, 'Do you think you don't remember them because they didn't disturb you?'"

I was not sure what the apparition meant, but I could guess. If Ruth had played with apparitions as a child, she had probably found them pleasant and undisturbing. Perhaps later she had learned to feel ashamed of having played with them and had wished to forget them. The childhood apparitions that she had told me about had visited her against her conscious will; in that sense they had not been her responsibility, and so perhaps she had allowed herself to remember them unashamedly.

Ruth looked toward me. "Are the things the apparition is saying really my own thoughts?"

"Maybe the apparition will explain," I said.

If the apparition's statements were really Ruth's thoughts, I was telling her to answer her own question.

Ruth turned her eyes back to where she had been seeing it. "She's still here . . . Now she's telling me, 'I think you are beautiful, for you are me.'"

In saying "you are me," the apparition seemed to be answering Ruth's question.

Ruth went on telling me what the apparition was saying. "'Go inside me and stay there until the present day. It's good for your research, and it won't frighten you. Believe that it's natural and not strange.'"

"Do you know," I asked Ruth, "what's meant by 'stay there until the present day'?"

"Yes, that I can go back in time to whatever part of my past I like, as long as it's before the present. I can't go beyond today into the future, into the part of my life I haven't yet lived."

"What's meant by 'Go inside me'?" I asked.

"I have to ask her . . . She's saying, 'Just relax and go into me . . . So long as we're joined, it's possible. You start at any age you choose, and go backward or forward . . . You haven't told Morty everything. Things will become apparent to him when the experiment is completed . . . Don't be afraid.'"

I supposed that the apparition was inviting Ruth to approach her and merge with her, as Ruth had done with her father's apparition.

Ruth looked at me. "The apparition has gone now," she said. "I'm shaky. My head hurts. I'm not sad, but I feel like crying. I'm sweating and feeling clammy, the way I often used to after making apparitions. I'd like a shower. My mouth is so dry. A lot of it is fear. The apparition said, 'Don't be afraid,' but I am frightened. I'm starving. Is it hunger or cowardice?"

I shrugged my shoulders.

"The next time I make an apparition of myself I'll try to be brave and go into her and travel back into my past. Do you think it'll be safe?"

"I don't see why not."

"That's a safe answer." She laughed.

"Tell me what part of my past I should return to," Ruth said to me the next time I saw her.

"Why don't you ask the apparition to tell you?"

Ruth stared into space for a moment. "There, she's here . . . She's saying it doesn't matter."

"Ask again."

Again Ruth stared. "The apparition said, 'Maybe you should go back to five years old . . . O.K. . . . It's as though I'm observing myself at five now . . . I can see the dress I'm wearing that day.

It's a little cotton dress. It was once white with a pattern of blue flowers, but now it's old, the white has gone gray, and the pattern has faded. The waist is gathered, and there are four buttons at the back. It's so short that it doesn't come down far enough to cover the bottom of my panties.

"It's early in the morning. I'm barefoot. I don't think my hair has been combed yet. There's grass in front of my house, and stickers in the grass. I've got one in my foot, and I'm getting it out. I'm thinking I'll be glad to be old enough to go to school. No one else is outside yet. I'm in the neighborhood alone. The sun feels good. I get some honeysuckle from a bush and chew on it. My mother sees me and yells at me not to eat it.

"I'm stepping up onto the porch. The concrete under my feet is hot. I'm entering the house. The door is green. It squeaks as it opens and closes. I go upstairs. The steps feel cold.

"Upstairs in my room is my plastic doll. The hair on her head doesn't feel like real hair—it's molded into her head. I'm talking to her, and she's talking to me. I'm her mummy, and she's my baby. I feel guilty because I've got another doll, a rag doll—she smiles on one side of her head and cries when you turn her head to the other side. I don't like her as much as the plastic doll. I think the rag doll knows I like the plastic doll more. I'm singing and talking to my plastic doll, telling her I love her and will buy her a brand-new outfit, because I've got a lot of money.

"Mallory, my sister, is coming upstairs. I can see her at that age. Her teeth seem too big for her face. She makes fun of me for talking to the doll. I feel ashamed. I put the doll down. I go to the bathroom and shut the door. I'm crying. I dry my face. The bottom of my foot is sore, and it stings. I check to see if the sticker made a hole in it. The door to the bathroom is shut. When it's shut, the fan in the window goes faster. The fan is making a loud noise. My mother shouts at me to open the door. I do, and go downstairs.

"Breakfast is ready. In the room are a green couch, a green chair, and a blond coffee table. The curtains are white and plastic, and you can see through them. I don't like them, because

I've seen them only in shanty houses. Everyone is talking. I can actually hear the voices. My brother, Andrew, wants some money for the movies—his class is going on Saturday at two. My mother says, 'Don't worry, I'll get money for you to go.' Mallory tells them about my talking to the doll. They laugh.

"My mother is shooing me out of the kitchen. She says to me that it's O.K., I can love my babies, but I shouldn't think they're real. She says I must stop talking to myself. I start to cry. I want my grandmother. My mother says I must stop that, that my grandmother is too old to look after me. My mother looks pretty to me. She's thin and has dark brown hair. She smiles a lot. I feel badly about my baby doll. I feel my mother has hurt its feelings. I go back upstairs to get it."

All this time Ruth had been staring straight ahead and had barely moved. Now she turned to me and relaxed in her chair. The experience was over.

She had evoked thoughts, sensations, colors, sounds, and voices as if they had been unfolding while she was speaking—though this had been a day twenty years ago.

"I can recall everything that just happened," she said. "At the start, I saw the apparition. Then I thought my way into her. As I did, I started seeing myself as a little girl and feeling the feelings I'd had then. Yet I still knew I was an adult sitting here talking to you.

"I brought to mind things I'd forgotten. Mallory's hair was a different color—a dirtier blond than it is now. It was also shorter and in a different style. I remember now that she used to wear it like that." Ruth took a deep breath. "I guess it was just an ordinary day—nothing important."

"I think it was a very interesting day, and relevant," I said. "Your experiencing apparitions as if they were real seems reminiscent of your talking to dolls as if they were real. Your thinking of yourself recently as crazy for experiencing apparitions could be related to Mallory's laughing at you and your mother's reproaching you then."

"Yes, I see that," she replied. "I remember now that I have had relationships with people who weren't really there. The people who caught me would tell tales about me, and I'd get ridiculed or spanked. My grandmother was the only one who didn't criticize me. She used to join in my doll games. Whenever my mother found me treating something imaginary as real, she'd scold me. If one of my children brought me an imaginary bird by cupping their hands, and said, 'Look at this, Ma,' I'd say, 'Where did you get it?' But if I'd done that with my mother, she'd have said, 'That's not real,' and I'd have felt ashamed."

I asked, "Do you believe you were reexperiencing an actual day from your past just now?"

"I think so. I'm going to phone my mother and ask her if she recalls that day."

"What will you ask her?"

"If she remembers Mallory making fun of me for talking to my dolls."

Ruth asked her mother about the event, and her mother said she remembered it.

"My mother said I used to talk to dolls, but didn't after that day. I think I went on talking to them until I was seven or eight, but was more careful after that day not to let anyone catch me. I'd hold one doll up to my ear, and it would whisper.

"My brother Andrew once tore a leg off one of my dolls. I thought the doll was crying, because of what he'd done. Everyone said it was just a doll, and I'd get another one. But I was brokenhearted.

"My mother told me something even more interesting. When I was two years old, I used to see people who weren't there. It scared everyone."

"Why were they scared?" I asked.

"I don't know. I didn't pursue the matter."

"If you did see people who weren't there, it may explain your apparition's remark a few days ago that you hadn't started seeing apparitions in the summer of 1976."

"Yes, that occurred to me too."

"I wonder if you ever had an imaginary companion as a child. Do you know what that is?"

"I think so. My son, George, used to have one. He'd call him Georgie. He thought of Georgie as if he was real. We'd always have to give Georgie a place at the table and put food on his plate. George let Georgie watch television and sit on a chair with him. He'd try to pick a chair large enough for both of them to sit in together. He may have had a sense of touching Georgie, because he'd sit with his arm around Georgie's back. They'd play together too. I tried to get him to show me where Georgie lived. He'd point up the street, but never showed me the particular house."

I nodded. "Thay's exactly what I meant by an imaginary companion."[22]

"I knew about Georgie only what my son told me. I never saw or heard Georgie myself. Georgie used to have some puppies that would visit him. Once, George let Georgie in through the back door while I was washing dishes. George announced that Georgie was here to play. I turned around, and said, 'That's nice.' George got upset, because when I'd turned around I'd stepped on the tail of one of the puppies.

"The last time I remember his seeing Georgie, we were parked in our car. It was raining. George said, 'Here's my friend Georgie.' I said, 'Let him in.' He said, 'He has to bring all his puppies in.' We opened the car door and let them all in. George had us move over to make room for everyone. Then he got angry at me about something. He took it out on Georgie, and said that Georgie's mother wanted him and that Georgie had to get out of our car.

"When I came back from the hospital after delivering Heather, Georgie had stopped coming to play with George. George would say, 'I wish Georgie would come to play with me.' I'd say, 'Why don't you invite him?' He'd say, 'Georgie's mother won't let him come over to our house anymore.' I don't think they played together after that.

"You don't think all this is hereditary, do you?" she asked.

"I don't know," I said. "George's imaginary companion and your apparitions may or may not be the same sort of phenomena. I do know that imaginary companions in children of George's age are common, whereas before meeting you I'd never heard of apparitions who came and went under an adult's control."

The next time Ruth and I were together, she took some time out to eat a cheese sandwich. "I feel guilty about wasting time eating," she said as she ate. "I'm going to make an apparition of myself and give her a bite, so that the sandwich will get eaten more quickly."

After a moment, she turned the uneaten part of the sandwich toward what I supposed was the apparition's mouth. "Here you go . . . taking my hand, and now taking a bite of the sandwich."

Ruth looked at me. "The apparition took a great big bite, and then backed away. I like sharing my sandwich with her."

"Tell her not to eat too quickly," I said, "or she'll get indigestion."

Ruth laughed.

"Let's have her take you into your past once more," I said.

"She hasn't finished eating yet."

I waited while Ruth ate the last of the sandwich.

"O.K., we're ready." Ruth stared at a space in front of her eyes. "Now I can see I'm at school. I'm in the fourth grade. Mrs. Green is my teacher. She's talking to us about God and about loving each other. I look around the room. Mrs. Green has arranged the seating so that all the rich kids are on one side by the window, and all the poor kids are by the wall. That's where I am. I'm unhappy today, because she's just moved two of my good friends to the other side of the room. I don't want to be on the side I'm sitting on.

"She's telling us the Bible story of Joseph's coat. Now she's telling me to pay attention and to stop daydreaming.

"I don't say anything.

"She says, 'Just say, "Yes, ma'am."'

"I still don't say anything.

"She says, 'Come up to the front of the room.'

"I'm embarrassed, and my face gets red. I see Johnny Mancuso laughing. I don't care about him laughing, because he gets into trouble all the time.

"She says, 'Say, "Yes, ma'am" and "I'm sorry."'

"I say nothing.

"She pinches my ear until it hurts.

"I think how much I hate her. I'll bet God doesn't like her either. Someone once told me that hypocrites get struck by lightning.

"She says I have to sit outside the class and won't be able to hear the Bible story. I'm pleased. I've got some chewing gum in my pocket that I'd chewed on the way to school and saved.

"I'm outside, in the hall. I hear Miss Moore, a teacher across the hall, doing something with flowers—each child is growing one. Mrs. Green is still talking about that stupid old coat. I'm wondering if I'll have to go to the principal's office.

"The bell rings. It's recess time. I ask Mrs. Green if I can go out.

"She says, 'No.'

"I thought she'd change her mind. But she made me sit in the coatroom. She's got a big sponge and she tells me to wash every desk and the blackboard.

"I say I won't.

"She says I will.

"I shake my head no and say I'm not the maid.

"She says if I don't, I'm not going to go out for any recesses or play periods again.

"I say I won't wash the desks. My grandma once told me that if you feel you're in the right, you shouldn't let anybody frighten you into backing down.

"Mrs. Green says I should return to my seat in the classroom. She gives me schoolwork to do. I can hear the children outside playing. I'm doing arithmetic. I can see the figures on the page. Forty-nine times twenty-three. Next is a problem for me to read. That's as far as I get. I'm looking out the window.

"Mrs. Green sits down in the desk in front of me. She asks me if I'd like her and her husband to pick me up and go with them to Sunday school.

"I tell her my momma doesn't allow us to go to Roly Holy churches. That's the kind of church she and her husband go to, where people shout and dance.

"She walks out. I feel badly about what I said to her. The children are walking back in.

"She didn't make me stay in all the time she'd said she would. The next play period, about noon, she let me go out to play."

Ruth's experience was over. "I don't see any significance in that day," she said.

She was Joseph in a way, I thought. He was a dreamer who was exiled for his dreams and sold into slavery. But later, he gained Pharaoh's favor and rose to prominence. When Ruth met me, she was feeling frightened she would be put away—exiled—in a mental ward. But through her dreaming or daydreaming, that is her experiencing apparitions, she had risen in importance. She was now a research subject and was receiving a lot of attention and interest.

I explained my thoughts to her.

"Yes, I see the connections," she said. "I like that."

I half-asked and half-asserted, "You think that what you just reported actually happened once in just that way?"

"I think so. It all seems very familiar to me."

I wondered if there was a way to verify her view, but I could think of none.

"How about calling these sessions memory trances?" she asked.

"O.K." I liked the expression, despite my uncertainty about whether her experiences were actual memories. "Can you say how you bring on a memory trance?"

"I produce an apparition of myself several feet away. Then she and I move toward each other. At some point I stop seeing her. There are no longer two of us. Then I start seeing some scene, such as myself as a girl in the fourth-grade classroom. When I first saw myself as a little girl just now, I felt numb and tingling all over. My tongue got thick and heavy, and my lips felt large. I felt as I did during the first dream I ever told you about, but this time the feelings were milder."

"How far back into my past do you think I can go in these memory trances?" Ruth asked me a few days later.

"You know whom to ask."

"At least you're different from most psychiatrists. I've heard that whenever you ask a psychiatrist something, he says, 'What do you think?' But you say, 'Ask the apparition.'"

I laughed.

"I'll have to bring her here again, I guess," Ruth said with a sigh, pretending to be exasperated. Ruth stared a moment. "She's here now. She's saying, 'You can become a baby again. You can go back to your mother's womb.'"

Ruth looked at me. "I'm astonished. It's hard to believe. What good will it do me if I can? A baby can't talk. Wouldn't it be degrading if I could only gurgle like a baby?"

"Ask the apparition," I said.

"Pretty soon she and I aren't going to need you anymore," she replied.

Her eyes turned toward the apparition. "I'll ask if I'd be able to talk to you . . . She says I could if I wasn't too young."

The apparition left.

Ruth turned toward me. "When I go back to infancy I'd like there to be only two parties in the room: me as an infant and you. I don't want me as an adult there. I want to lose all consciousness of my adult self."

When Ruth next tried a memory trance, she saw herself as an infant sitting on her family's porch.

She did not talk during the trance, but told me afterward what had happened.

"Comparing the infant's size with my own kids' size at different ages," Ruth said, "I'd guess she was about twelve months old."

The infant had walked across the porch to a swing and tried to climb up on it, but the swing had flown back and hit her on the chin, making her bleed.

"I felt the blood and pain on my chin," Ruth said. "However, I couldn't forget about myself at the age I am now. I couldn't lose myself."

Possibly, the incident with the swing had actually occurred. Perhaps some time afterward someone had told her of it, and she was reliving in the memory trance what she remembered having been told.

I noted that blood and pain, which were frequent intruders into her life, had invaded this very early memory.

"I'd like to try going right back to my mother's womb," Ruth said to me the next day. "Last night I tried it on my own a few times, and almost did it."

After initially staring at what I supposed was the apparition of herself, she closed her eyes.

She sat silently with eyes closed for about two minutes.

Then she opened them and sighed. "Wow!" she said.

"Yes?"

"I think I did it. I was in her womb. I didn't see anything. It was hot—not warm and not burning hot—but hot. Then labor began—I think that's what it was. It didn't feel good. My head was really hurting. The pain was in my head, nowhere else.

"I'm so tired. It wasn't an enjoyable experience at all. My head still hurts.

"Being in the womb before labor began was almost too sweet to talk about. I think there's a connection between that feeling and the feeling just after sexual intercourse."

This last memory trance fascinated me. Was Ruth remembering here an actual experience from her own past? I am aware that some people—including a few psychiatrists—believe it is possible for an adult to recollect prebirth or birth experiences.[23] However, as far as I knew, it had not been proved that any human being had done so. If I could have obtained evidence about her birth and her mother's pregnancy from someone else or from hospital records, I could have compared that evidence with further experiences of going back to the womb that I would have urged her to have. But no other evidence was available.

That was the last memory trance we did while Ruth was still living in England.

When she returned to England a year later, she said she had brought about memory trances many times during the year, alone or with Paul, and had found she no longer needed to use the apparition of herself.

"I can tell you how I do it, but only up to a point, not completely. Say I want to return to six years old. I sit and relax. I picture a particular day when I was six. I remember many days from then, though not all of them. I see what I was doing that day and center my thoughts on it. I concentrate really hard on seeing myself on that day, and I gradually begin to feel my feelings on that day, and I get deeper and deeper, and then . . . that's all I can describe. After that I don't know how I feel."

"Do you do it with your eyes open or closed?"

"Closed, when I'm going into it. It's easier that way. When I come out of it, it's like waking up in the morning."

Upon emerging from the trances she had been having recently, she had found she could recall little or nothing of what had transpired during them. When Paul had been with her, she had needed to rely on him to tell her. When she had been on her own, she had been unable to retrieve anything. Consequently she had lost interest in bringing on the trances.

She did not understand—nor did I—why amnesia for these sessions had been occurring. "It seems that when it works best," she said, "I don't remember it."

"Would you like to do some trances with me?"

"I guess so, but only if you'll tell me afterward what happened."

"It's a deal!"

I wanted to try to explore in the trances her make-believe experiences as a small child, such as daydreaming, imaginary companions, and dramatic play.

"Why don't you try returning to six years old?" I said.

"All right."

We were sitting in my office. She relaxed in her chair and closed her eyes. "I'm beginning to feel funny. It's happening."

After a little over a minute, she opened her eyes and looked at me. She looked around the room and then at me again. I decided to break the silence. "Hello."

She put the knuckle of her left thumb in her mouth and sucked it while lowering her head. It was a child's gesture and was uncharacteristic of the Ruth I knew.

"What's your name?" she asked, sucking her thumb. It was Ruth's voice, but weaker and higher-pitched than usual. I recognized that as a child she could not have known my name, as she had not yet met me.

"Morty. What's yours?" I said.

"Cheepy."

I decided to get right to the point. "I'm very interested in children who've seen ghosts or people who weren't really there. I think children can sometimes see people who aren't there much better than grown-ups can. I'd like to know if you've ever seen somebody who wasn't there. I don't mean in a dream. I mean awake and with your eyes open."

She looked at my books on the wall behind her. "You've got a lot of books. Do they have pictures in them?" The thumb left her mouth.

"Some of them do."

"Any pictures of trees?" She was looking at me.

"Yes, why do you ask about trees?"

"I don't know."

"Well, are you going to tell me?"

"What?"

"If you've ever seen anybody who wasn't really there."

She looked at her lap, where her fingers were fidgeting. "You can't do that."

"Some people can."

"My momma says no."

"Did you ask your momma about it?"

She shook her head no. "If you see somebody, then they're there."

"How about when you were a little girl, younger than you are now? Did you see anyone then?"

She was silent for a moment. "You're nosy," she said.

I laughed.

"You know what I'm supposed to say?" she said.

"What?"

"Go ask my momma."

"Does your momma know?"

"She told me when anybody asked me questions, I should tell them to go ask her."

"But how can I find out from her if she doesn't know?"

"Then it's a secret."

"Let me ask you . . ."

"I can draw."

"Yes?"

"Could I draw a picture for you?"

I gave her a pencil and a pad of blank paper.

On the paper she drew a flower.

"Look at my flower," she said.

"It's nice. When you were a little girl, two or three or four, did you ever see anybody that other people couldn't see?"

"I don't really like you," she said. I thought I detected a coy smile.

"Why is that?" I asked.

"'Cause you ask too many questions."

"But you give me such interesting answers."

"Well, it's hard to be nice to grown-up people when you're not supposed to tell them, and it's none of their business."

"I'm not going to get you into trouble. Did you ever see anybody?"

"You won't tell?"

"I won't."

"Well, if you do, I'm not talking to you anymore."

"O.K."

"Sometimes I do, when I want to."

"Whom do you see, when you want to?"

"Friends. And sometimes I see my uncles."

"Are they really there? Do other people see them?" I remembered that Daniel, my son, had said at five or six: "If one person sees a ghost, it's not real. If two people see it, it's real."

She said, "I don't let anyone see them."

"Can you tell me about the last time that happened?"

"I saw my Uncle Al. We played jacks."

"Could anyone else see him?"

"I was hiding."

"If someone else had been there, would they have seen him?"

"I'm not a witch."

"I know. Have you ever done that with anyone besides Al?"

She nodded yes.

"With whom else?"

"When I had measles, I saw everybody."

"How old were you then?"

"Three. Maybe three. I was little."

"Whom did you see?"

"I saw my momma, and I saw my grandma, and I saw that uncle, and I saw a princess, and I saw all my friends."

"All at the same time?"

"All at one time."

She was recalling something which she had not remembered as an adult. A child of six can recall events from three that an adult cannot, I thought.

"Did you talk to them?" I asked. "And did they talk back?"

"My momma says when you daydream, they don't really talk back. You just pretend they do."

"How did it feel to you? Did you like it? Was it fun?"

She nodded. "It scares my momma."

"How does she know about it?"

"Sometimes she hears me. . . . When I'm not careful."

"Whom do you talk to?"

"I've got three friends I talk to a lot."

"Yes? What are their names?"

"You promise not to tell?"

"I promise. It's just between us."

She lowered her voice. "One's name is Linda, and another one's name is Margaret, and then there's Eddie. And all my friends have got black hair."

"Do your friends all come at once or only one at a time?"

"However many I want."

"Have they been your friends for a long time?"

"Eddie has."

"For how long?"

"For years."

She could have meant "for" or "four" years. "What's he like?"

"He's just like me, except he's a boy. And he don't fight."

"Does your momma know about Eddie?"

"No, and you'd better not tell her."

"I'm not going to tell anybody, until you're grown up. I'll keep it secret until then."

"You won't know me then."

"We might meet again someday."

"My grandma knows my secret."

"She knows about your friends?"

"She knows all my secrets, and she tells me all of her secrets. And when I grow up, I'm going to buy a big house, and it's gonna have an elevator, so my grandma won't have to walk upstairs when her feet hurt, and I'm going to be her doctor so I can always take care of her, and I'm gonna have lots of money."

"I hope you do. All right, I'd like you to grow up now, and come back." As I said that, I got up from my chair, walked over to Ruth, and touched her hand. I hoped and expected that this would end her trance, though I fleetingly worried, What if her trance doesn't end? . . . What then? Within a few seconds Ruth had returned to her normal state.

"What do you remember about the end of your experience just now?" I asked.

"Feeling tingling, then seeing your books, and then gradually back to normal. I feel as if I've been dreaming, but couldn't remember any of it."

In the memory trances I had seen her undergo earlier, she had seen and experienced herself as a little girl, but had remained aware of being an adult. This time she displayed no such awareness and she talked to me as if she were actually a child. She also sucked her thumb as a child of six might. Perhaps her apparent unawareness of her adult self during this trance was related to her later amnesia about the content of the trance.

I read my notes of the trance to her. She thought that the events sounded familiar, but she could not have brought any of them to mind herself.

I read to her about her as a girl asking me if my books had any pictures of trees in them.

"I recollect now that I knew why I was asking," Ruth commented, "but I didn't want you to know. I was thinking of trees in woods—and woods are where I'd played with ghosts."

"You've never told me about playing with ghosts in woods."

"I never remembered before. The little girl was thinking about the ghosts in the woods. That's how I've remembered them."

I continued reciting my notes.

"I remember that when I mentioned playing jacks with my Uncle Al," she said, "I was referring to an apparition of him. I'd forgotten all about that experience until this session."

I reached the part about her measles when she was three years old.

"When I was in the children's home," she said, "I had measles, mumps, and chicken pox all about the same time. Before I could get over one, I'd get the other. I was in the home's hospital. I'd forgotten the bit about inventing people then to comfort myself. I remember it now for the first time."

"Were the people you invented apparitions?"

"I can't remember if they looked real and fleshy. They might have been creatures that I imagined, not apparitions. But they seemed real to me then."

She referred to her three friends, Linda, Margaret, and Eddie, as imaginary playmates. She could recall what each of them had looked like, but not if she had ever actually seen them. If she had not seen them, they may have been imaginary playmates of the sort that many young children have.

Ruth and I were sitting in my office. I recalled the man in the white top whom she had seen one night at the foot of her bed before she was four, and whom she had seen on three consecutive nights at nine, and once more at sixteen.

"How about going back to the morning after you'd first seen that man by your bed in the children's home?" I said.

"All right. After I'd seen him that night, I'd gone into Big Mama's bed to sleep . . . O.K., I'm starting to concentrate." She closed her eyes.

After about a minute her eyes opened, and she looked at me.

"Hello, Ruth."

"Where's Miss Sanders?" She began to suck her left thumb. She looked frightened.

"I don't know," I said. "How are you this morning?"

"Who are you?"

"My name's Morty."

She had met me in her last memory trance, when she had allegedly been six, but she couldn't remember me from that trance, I reckoned, since she was now supposedly younger than four; how could she recognize someone whom she had not met before?

"Have you ever seen me before?" I asked.

She continued sucking her thumb and said nothing. "Where's Miss Sanders?" she asked again.

I guessed that "Miss Sanders" was Big Mama's name. "Did you sleep with her last night?" I asked.

She nodded yes.

"I don't know where she is," I said. "Why did you sleep with her?"

She furrowed her brows, trembled, and sucked her thumb more vigorously. "Are you in my dream?"

"No," I replied.

She sniffled.

"Did you have a dream last night?" I asked.

She nodded. "Are you a mean man?"

"No. Could you tell me your dream?"

"He wouldn't go away." She whimpered as she said it, and went on sucking her thumb.

"Who wouldn't?"

"That big man."

"What big man?"

"That one when I called my grandma."

"Why did you call your grandma?"

"'Cause he was there. I don't like him."

"Why?"

"I don't know. Why did he come last night? Was he going to get me? Was he going to get me?"

"Did you think he was?"

She nodded.

"What's his name?"

"He don't got one." Her thumb went deeper into her mouth.

"Have you ever seen him before, when you weren't in bed?"

She nodded.

"Where?"

She went on sucking and said nothing.

"Where?"

"At that woman's house."

"What's that woman's name?"

"I don't know."

"When was it?"

"There was a wooden fence and a gate . . . I want my grandma." She whimpered again. "Do you know where my grandma lives?"

"I could find out."

"Will you go tell her I want her?"

"I'll see. Was that the only other time you saw him?"

She nodded. "We walked there. My momma carried me."

"Did your momma know that man?"

"I don't know."

"When you saw him that time when your momma carried you, were you afraid of him?"

"He didn't talk to me."

"Whom did he talk to?"

"My momma."

"Do you remember anything he said?"

She shook her head no.

"Do you remember anything your momma said to him?"

"I want my grandma, please."

"Are you scared?"

She nodded.

She had once told me, I recalled, that when he had first appeared at the foot of her bed, the white top he had been wearing had reminded her of a doctor's top. "Is he a doctor?" I asked.

She nodded. "I think."

"Was your mother going to him for help?"

"Where did he go?"

"Do you mean last night?"

She nodded.

"I don't know. What did you do at that house with the wooden fence and the gate?"

"We sleeped there."

"Overnight?"

She nodded.

"Did you sleep in the same room as your momma?"

She shook her head no.

"Did your momma sleep in the same room as that man?"

Again she shook her head. "That man leave."

"Where did he go?"

"I don't know. Will he get me?"

"I don't think so. I think you're quite safe here."

"I want my grandma. It was dark." She clutched the collar of her blouse and put it into her mouth.

As the same apparition had manifested to Ruth again at nine and at sixteen—at older ages than the one at which she was presently portraying herself—I wanted to see if she would display awareness of those later experiences. "Do you think you'll ever see that man again?" I asked.

"I don't want to."

"How about when you get bigger than you are now?"

She shook her head no.

"How are you feeling now?"

"I'll be good if you get my grandma."

I recalled her from her trance in the same way as I had the previous time. Again she returned in a moment to her ordinary state. And again she was amnesic for what had been occurring.

I read my notes of the session to her. She found it exciting that she had remembered in the trance having seen that man once before in nonapparitional form. While in her ordinary mental state, she had tried and failed many times to recall some such memory.

"I can see that whole scene now," she said. "I'm remembering it for the first time. I think I was about two years old when I saw the man at the woman's house."

As in the previous return to childhood in a trance, she was recalling something which apparently had happened even earlier in childhood and which she had had no memory of as an adult.

"That woman had dark circles under her eyes," she said. "She came and got me, Mallory, Andrew, and my mother. Everyone was upset. The woman was good to us, but her looks frightened me. We and that woman were walking at night. I was in my mother's arms, and then she passed me to that woman. I was old enough to walk. They were carrying me to get there faster, and they were getting tired. I can feel now what it was like to be carried in their arms, the jogging in their arms.

"We crossed a street, and on a corner was a house. It had a

wooden fence with slats running up and down and a half-open gate. Stairs went up to a wooden porch with rocking chairs on it. I can see that house, and most of all that gate.

"In the house this man, and my mother, and that woman were talking. I wasn't listening. I was busy playing—with Andrew, I think. The man and my mother walked out onto the porch, talking. Then he left.

"We spent the night there. Andrew, Mallory, and I slept in the same bed. It was a spookish kind of night, because I knew something was going on. Something seemed wrong. It was the same kind of night on which I later saw the man's apparition—black and dark.

"Whatever was happening that night disturbed me. I didn't know what it was then, and I still don't. It's been kept from me. I'm going to ask my mother who that man was. I'm sure she knows. But she'll probably say she doesn't remember, even if she does."

Some weeks later Ruth asked her mother, but as Ruth had expected, her mother said she did not know.

Had Ruth really seen the man at two years old? She thought that she had, and that the scene she recalled in the trance had once actually occurred. Without corroboration from someone else who had been there at the time, I could not feel sure.

Except perhaps for the standard intelligence test, the Rorschach or inkblot test has been the most frequently used test in clinical psychology. Its standard set of ten inkblots, reproduced on cards, serve as stimuli for the subject's associations. I wanted to see how Ruth would respond to the inkblots, both in her normal state and then in memory trances, to see whether her associations to the same inkblot would be similar or different, and how her responses in the trances would compare with those of children at corresponding ages. I also hoped that the testing would add to Ruth's understanding of herself.

Anne Kilcoyne is a clinical psychologist who has worked in London at the Tavistock Clinic and at the Middlesex Hospital.

She is also a practitioner of psychotherapy and a qualified teacher. Before meeting Ruth, she had given the inkblot test to many adults, adolescents, and children, but never to an adult who had returned to childhood.[24]

I spent a few minutes telling Anne about Ruth, including the father's attack upon her at ten, her experiences of being persecuted by her father's apparition, the method of therapy I had used, and some of the experiments we had done.

In talking with Anne, I referred to Ruth as Muriel. This was the name that Ruth and I had agreed she would be known by to all research workers. We gave them a false name because Ruth did not want them to connect her real name with her childhood history, which she knew I might need to tell them. For the reader's convenience I continue to call her Ruth.

Anne was seven and a half months pregnant when she tested Ruth, and her belly was obviously swollen. I mention this because her pregnancy was referred to during the testing.

Anne had not met Ruth before testing her and chatted with her in a room in my house to get acquainted. Anne wanted to remain alone with Ruth when Ruth took the test in her normal state.

Anne told me later what had ensued.

They had sat at a desk in the room. "I'm going to be showing you some cards one at a time," Anne had said. "On each card you'll see a design made by an inkblot. I'd like you to look at each card carefully and tell me anything it looks like or reminds you of. Take as long as you like. There are no right or wrong answers. No two people see exactly the same thing. Just be sure to tell me all that you see."

Ruth responded to each of the ten inkblots, and Anne recorded the responses.

When Ruth finished the test, they invited me into the room.

Anne and Ruth now sat side by side, and I sat opposite them.

I suggested that Ruth respond in memory trances at seven, ten, and fifteen to three or four inkblots, the same ones each time.

She agreed. "At seven, I'd like it to be before my father came to live with us," she said. "That would keep it from being too unpleasant."

She closed her eyes and covered her face with a hand. After sitting stiffly immobile for about a minute, she opened her eyes and relaxed her body. I assumed that she was in a memory trance.

"I wonder if you could look at some cards and tell us what you see on them," I said.

"O.K." said Ruth.

Anne handed her card VI from the standard Rorschach set of inkblots.

Ruth looked at it. "I see a train up here going down this railroad track. And this is the engine. And it's a big train with wings, and it can fly. And it's got lots and lots of smoke coming out of the back of the engine car that's making a big ball of smoke over the whole train."

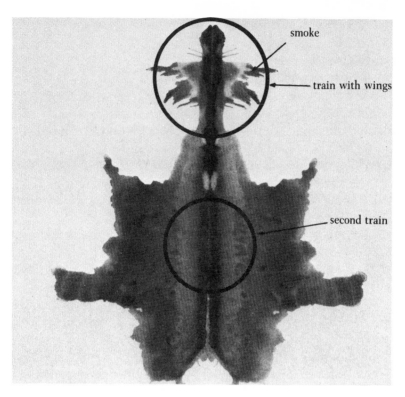

I have indicated on the facsimile of the inkblot where she saw various things.

She saw a second train lower on the inkblot. "That train's going a different way, and that train is going that way. But they was going to be together, but then they stopped being together. That's why there's lots of smoke, because there's two trains. But this train don't go as fast because it don't have wings. I don't want to do this no more."

"This card or this activity?" asked Anne.

"Are we playing?"

"It's a bit like a game."

"I'll play."

"Why did you say you wanted to stop? You didn't like this card?"

"There's nobody on the train eating ice cream or nothing."

"The two trains had been going in the same direction. Why did they decide to separate?"

"Because they didn't like each other."

"Why didn't they?"

"Because that train that can fly, there's a bad man on that train and that's his train. He said he'd like to have his own train. I don't know. They just don't like each other."

"Which train would you like to be on?"

"Not that one," she said, pointing to the train that could fly, "and this one maybe, just maybe this one," pointing to the other train.

"You're not keen on either of these trains. Where would you like to be?"

"In school."

"Why aren't you in school?"

"Because it's summertime," she said scornfully. "But I'm going to start school in the second grade, and then I won't have Mrs. Mason."

"What's she like?"

"She's mean. She won't let me go to the bathroom or let me get a drink of water because she's mean."

It is easy to see Ruth's two trains corresponding to her parents, who had separated, and the bad man's train that can fly corresponding to her father, who had left the family and been in jail before returning to the family. Whether it is too easy, which implies that Ruth was deliberately acting the part of herself at seven, I do not know. If she was enacting a role, she was doing it so competently that I did not feel at the time that she was doing so. She could not have rehearsed her answers, as she had not known in advance that she would be taking an inkblot test or would be taking it in memory trances.

Anne handed her card IV. "See what games you can play with this one," Anne said.

"That looks kind of like a clown, don't it?" Ruth said. "And he's making lots of people laugh. He's got two big black shoes on that's too big, and he's sitting on top of a barrel. He looks scary, but he's not scaring me. He's just something to laugh at. He's a good clown. He's got on a mask."

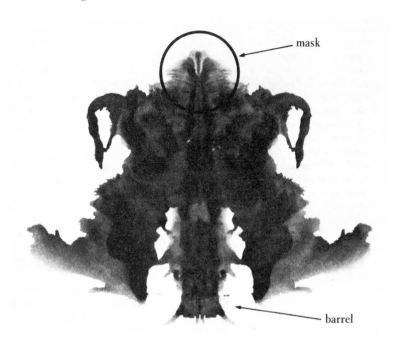

mask

barrel

"How does he make people laugh?" asked Anne.

"He gets in an itty-bitty barrel, and he rolls around all over the place. He wouldn't be able to get out of the barrel if he were really that fat, but he's not that fat."

"Does he remind you of any man you know?"

"I know one," Ruth replied.

"Who?"

"I'm not going to tell you."

"Why not? Is he a secret?"

Ruth nodded. "But he's not scary. He's a nice man."

"Does he like you?"

Ruth nodded.

"Does he like your mother?"

"I don't know. Maybe he don't know her. I've got a pretty mama."

"Have you? What does she look like?"

"She's the prettiest mama in the whole school. She's big, she's got long hair, and she's got big pretty teeth that shine, and she's got pretty dresses."

"What's your daddy like?"

"Which one?"

"I didn't know you had more than one. Have you?"

"I got lots of them, sort of. I do got one. I bet you think I don't, but I do." Ruth began to cry. Tears dripped down her cheeks. "I got the best one."

"What's he like?"

"He's pretty. My grandma told me I got the prettiest daddy in the whole wide world and not to believe people like you. I mustn't believe people who say I don't have a daddy."

"But I didn't say that."

"I've got three. I'll bet you don't have three."

"Who are your three? Have they got names?"

"Yeah, but I'm not going to tell you."

Anne handed her card VII.

"This is a rocking horse," Ruth said. "And there's two rocking

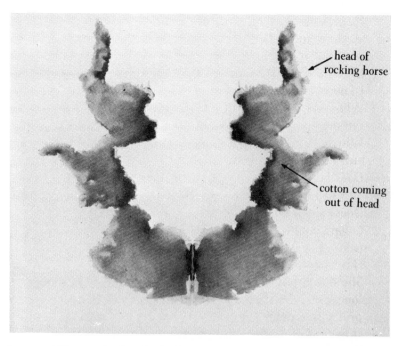

head of
rocking horse

cotton coming
out of head

horses. This is the head of a horse. You can sit on it, and you can rock back and forth."

"Would you like to rock on it?"

"I'm too big. It's for babies. And the cotton is coming out of the head, just here. Someone bit it on the ear, and all the cotton is coming out. A baby bit it. I bit Duncan."

"What did you bite him for?"

"Because he stuck my brother's domino in his pocket, so I bit him on the finger. Duncan made me mad, but I'm not going to bite anyone else, never. It's not nice to bite your friends. You don't have good pictures."

"No, they're not the best pictures in the world."

"Why don't you color them?"

"Here's a colored one." Anne showed her card VIII.

"That's a dumb picture," Ruth said.

"Thank you for looking at the cards for me."

"What's your name?"

"Anne, what's yours?"

"Cheepy."

I signaled to Ruth to emerge from the trance. When she did, she remembered nothing.

I had chosen age ten for Ruth's next memory trance to see how she would respond to the same inkblots after her father's assault. "How about two weeks after your father's assault?" I suggested to her.

"You wouldn't want me to make it then," she said, "because I was spending most of my time in bed. I was being accused of lying and of being crazy."

"When would you propose making it?" I asked her.

"Six weeks after."

While entering the trance, she behaved as she had while entering the previous one. Later she told us she had brought on the trance by concentrating upon an image of her baby sister, who had been born some hours before the assault, at six weeks old, and upon herself getting the baby a bottle.

When Ruth opened her eyes indicating she was in the trance, she looked at me and then at Anne. "I don't like him," she said to Anne. "He's not supposed to be here."

"Why don't you like him?" asked Anne.

"I just don't. Ask him to move farther away."

I moved the chair I was sitting on back a few feet.

"Do you know Judge Shelley?" Ruth asked Anne.

"No, who's he?"

"He's going to be in charge." Ruth was referring to the probate judge who would be in charge of her, she told us later.

"What do you need a judge for?" asked Anne.

"It's not nice to talk about. If you knew, you'd know. And if you don't know, you're not supposed to know. Are you here about that?"

"In a way. I'll be wanting you to look at some cards."

"Do you know him?"

"No."

"He'll be mad at you if you know."

Anne guessed Ruth was now talking about her father.

"I won't tell your father anything you tell me," Anne said.

"My momma told him."

"What did she say?"

"'Did you really?' she asked him."

"What did he say?"

"He said he didn't."

"Whom does your mother believe?"

"About what?"

"That it happened."

"I don't know what you're talking about."

"It seems as if you're frightened of talking to me. Whom do you like talking to?"

"Nobody. Are you a doctor?"

"Sort of."

"Are you a nurse?"

"No. I'm a psychologist."

"What's that?"

"It's a mind doctor. Would you like to see a doctor?"

"No. I don't want to see nobody."

"What have you been doing?"

"I get the baby a bottle sometimes, and I play, and I go out sometimes."

"What's the baby's name?"

Ruth gave her sister's real name.

"What's she like?"

"She's not so pretty. She looks like a warthog. She'll be pretty though." Later, when I read back my notes of this conversation to Ruth, she did not know what a warthog is or remember ever having used the word.

"Is your daddy still living at home?" asked Anne.

"Yeah. He's going to go away."

"Are you glad about that?"

Ruth nodded. "If he goes away, I hope he'll die. If I hope it hard enough, will it happen?"

"I don't know. Are you frightened he'll do it again?"

"He better not, or I'll run away."

"Where would you go?"

"I want to be a doctor's little girl."

"You want someone to look after you whom you'll feel safe with."

"No, I can look after myself. I'll go somewhere for a while, and then I'm going to run away and run away again and again and again."

"Why will you be running?"

"Because I'm big enough. Why do you want to know?"

"I'm interested in understanding how you're feeling."

"Do you have any girls?"

"No. I have a baby inside me. I don't know if it's a boy or a girl."

"You better not let it come out."

"Why? Do you think if a baby comes out, something bad will happen?"

"I don't know. Would you want to have a big girl?"

"You mean like you?"

"Yes."

"I'd like to have a girl like you. Would you like to be my girl?"

Ruth cried, and tears dripped down her cheeks.

"What does your grandmother say about what's been going on?"

"She told me not to tell nobody else, but she says I should tell the police and they'll see he never does it again. But I couldn't do that, because then they'd know about me."

"What would they know about you?"

Ruth said nothing.

"They'd know you did it too?"

"I'm not supposed to talk to you because I'll get in trouble."

"I won't tell anyone."

"He'll want to know where I've been."

"Who? Your father?"

"Yeah. He'll know if I tell a lie."

"Let's look at these cards. That way you'll have something to tell your father. You'll be able to say you were looking at picture cards."

"I'll still be in trouble."

"I'll have a word with your father and tell him not to get angry."

"Don't do that."

"Even if I say you were only looking at picture cards?"

"Yes."

Handing Ruth card IV, Anne explained what the cards were and what she wanted of her.

Ruth looked at it. "I see dark spots and light gray spots."

"Anything else?"

"Something stuck on a pole, but I don't know what it is."

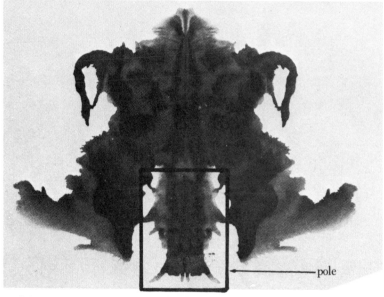

"Can you see anything else there?"

"No."

"Are you sure?"

"I said, 'No.'"
"You don't like that card, do you?"
Ruth shook her head no.
"Do you know what you don't like about it?"
"I don't want to talk about it."
Anne showed her card VII.

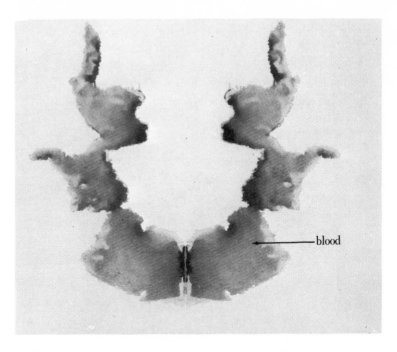

"What does that look like to you?" Anne asked.
"Babies."
"How many?"
"Two."
"Where are the heads?"
Ruth showed her.
"What's this part?"
"The baby's chest. There's blood there." Ruth pointed out where.

"Why is there blood there?" asked Anne.

"I don't know. The baby's just been born. Do babies bleed?"

"Sometimes, if they get cut."

"That's why the baby's bleeding, because someone got hurt. Are those babies bleeding?"

"They are if you say they are. Does it worry you that they're bleeding?"

"I don't care. I don't like babies."

Anne showed her card VI.

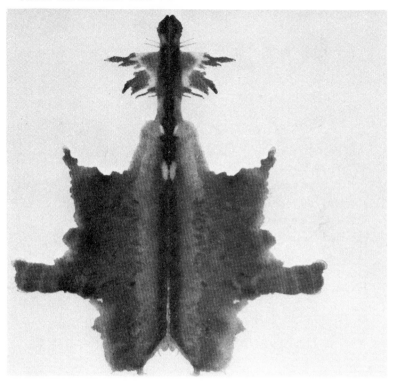

Ruth looked at it and began to cry. "I don't like it."

"Which part don't you like?"

"None of it."

"You want me to take it away."

Ruth nodded. "Why are you showing me bad pictures?"

"I didn't think it was bad. Why was it bad?"

Ruth did not answer.

"Which is the worst picture of the ones I showed you?" asked Anne, and she laid out cards IV, VI, and VII.

Ruth turned card VI facedown.

It was the same card on which she had seen two trains in the trance at seven.

"O.K. I'll keep that card covered up," said Anne, and she put it away.

"I'm going to be in trouble," said Ruth.

"I think we can keep our secret."

"Promise you won't tell him."

"I promise. Don't worry, you can tell your father you've been having a nap. I think we should finish."

"I feel sick. I've got flu."

"Maybe you should go and see Dr. Schatzman."

"Who?"

"Dr. Schatzman."

"Who's he?"

"He's a good person to see when you've been feeling as you feel. Would you like me to take you to him?"

"What will he do?"

"He'll try to make you feel better."

"I feel really sick. We through?"

Anne nodded.

"It's over now," I said to Ruth. "Come back now."

The trance ended.

"I'm feeling drained, and my body aches," Ruth said, "as if someone had just beaten me up."

"You were so scared during that trance," Anne said, "that you wouldn't even look at me."

Again Ruth remembered nothing of it.

This time, we took a half-hour coffee break before resuming work.

With eyes closed, Ruth now concentrated on entering a

memory trance, at fifteen. When she opened them, she seemed to
be in a trance.

"How are you?" Anne asked her.

"Fine," was her reply.

"My name's Anne."

"So?"

"So, I'm just introducing myself."

Ruth gave her real first name, not a pseudonym.

"I'm a psychologist. I think I should say that."

Ruth frowned. "Ach," she said in disgust.

"I'm sorry about that," Anne said.

"Is that your secretary?" Ruth asked, pointing at me sitting
across the room taking notes.

"Yes," Anne replied. "At least for this afternoon. Have you met
him before?"

"No. You should pay him more money."

"Why?"

"So he can buy himself some shoes."

I was wearing some cheap, shabby tennis shoes.

Anne laughed. "So, where are we now?" she asked.

"You're the psychologist, and you don't know where we are?"
Ruth looked around the room and furrowed her brow. "Where are
we?" She seemed genuinely puzzled.

"Do you recognize this place?" Anne asked.

Ruth shrugged her shoulders. "How long have I been here?"

"Since this morning," Anne replied.

"I was supposed to be going swimming at the coast this
afternoon. I don't know where I'm at." When I later read back the
conversation to Ruth, she recalled having been confused at this
point, since she had had in mind that the girls from the institution
had been scheduled to go swimming that afternoon.

"I guess you like hearing that I don't know where I'm at," Ruth
said.

"Why should I like that?"

"Most psychologists do, don't they?"

"I get the feeling you don't like psychologists."

"How did you ever guess?"

"I'd like you to look at some tests. No, 'tests' isn't the right word, because there are no grades. They're just splotches for you to see things in."

"To see if I'm crazy?"

"To see how you tick."

"That's what I meant."

Anne handed her card IV. "That's the first one," she said.

Ruth glanced at it. "I see snakes."

"Anything else?"

She looked at it a little longer. "Mmm. No."

"Where are the snakes?"

"All over it."

"Show me," Anne said.

Ruth flicked her fingers over different areas of the inkblot. "There, and there, and there, and there. Don't you see them?"

"No. Show me exactly where the snakes are."

Again Ruth flicked her fingers over different areas.

"Can you actually show me where the snakes are?"

"Aren't you supposed to say whatever you see?"

"I think you're fighting me. Let's talk about what you're really fighting about, so you can stop fighting."

"Your dumb pictures aren't going to tell you how I tick. Only I could tell you. That's the only way anyone could tell you."

"I agree," said Anne. "You tell me."

"I don't want to. Do you want me to tell you what I see on the card?" [See facing page.]

"Yes."

"It's an inkblot."

"It is. But what does it look like or remind you of?"

"A blob," said Ruth.

"A blob of what?"

"Measles and freckles."

Anne made some notes.

"I don't know what you're writing for," Ruth said. "You've got a

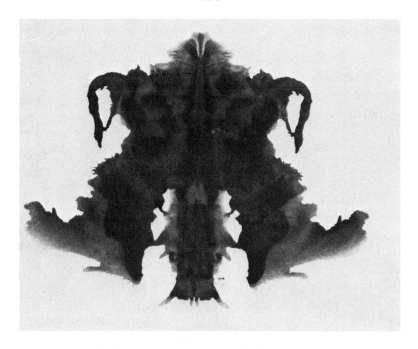

secretary." She flung a contemptuous look at me.

"I like to make my own records," Anne said. "Show me where you can see the measles and freckles."

Ruth showed her.

"Yes, I see the spots," Anne said.

"You're a psychologist, and you see spots?" Ruth whistled and looked at the ceiling in mock amazement.

"How about this one?" Anne said, handing her card VII.

"You tell me what you want me to say, and I'll say it," Ruth said.

"I don't have a ready-made formula."

"What do crazy people say?"

"Many different kinds of things. It depends on the particular way in which they're crazy."

"When Billy and I went to see the psychologist, we said we felt snakes crawling all up our legs. We went in one right after the other. We'd decided to pretend we were afraid of snakes. They were wrapped around our legs and out the windows. The psychologist looked so dumb, and didn't catch on."

"Were you putting me on when you said you saw snakes?"

"I wouldn't say that."

"All right, what about this card?"

"What does it matter what I say about some ink that someone spilled on paper? What do you want me to do this for? Are you doing some kind of survey?"

"Yes, sort of."

"Who are you comparing me to?"

"This particular survey is on you."

"Do you enjoy doing this?"

"Sometimes. If the other person does."

"Don't count on me. If I don't enjoy it, then you don't, and I'm not going to, so why are you doing it?"

"I'm a trier."

"I don't mean to be a bitch, but I just don't like none of this."

"What do you think is the point of this testing?" Anne asked.

"To give bored grown-ups something to do." She looked at me. "You got to keep confidential what we say in here," she said to Anne. "But what about him?"

"He's bound by the same rule, unless you give him your permission."

"I'm not giving him anything. Make sure he keeps anything I say away from Miss Finch."

"Who's she?"

"She's my social worker. She looks like a bullfrog. Her head looks like the head of a frog, her back splits at the bottom, she doesn't have any butt, and her legs are this thick." Ruth made a circle with her thumb and first finger. "I always expect her to say 'ribit.'"

"What does 'ribit' mean?"

"What a frog says. Where are you from?" she asked Anne.

"England."

"When are you going back?"

"Very soon," Anne said.

"Good."

"Why is that good?"

Ruth shrugged her shoulders. "Take it any way you want to."

"There's only one way to take it," Anne said.

"You got it," Ruth replied.

Ruth looked at the card.

"I see two old women, and a vagina," she said.

"Where are the two old women?"

Ruth showed her.

"What makes you think the women are old?" Anne asked.

"Their chins and noses are close together, like with old women."

"And where's the vagina?"

"You want me to point to it?" She seemed embarrassed.

Anne nodded.

Ruth pointed.

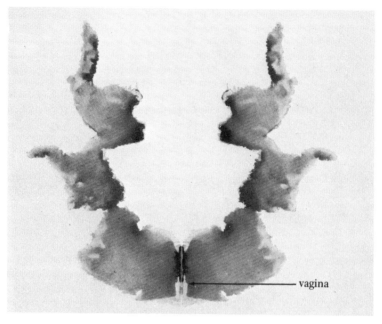

"I'm sorry," Anne said. "I can see it's difficult for you."

"If I don't cooperate, you'll tell the head, and she'll put me on restriction."

"I won't. It sounds like they don't understand you here."

"They're just here to make money. And we've got to be here because we don't have no other place to go. So you can't expect us to like them. They don't understand nothing. I didn't have a choice to come here for this, and you did."

"You could've pretended to have flu."

"Then I couldn't have done anything else all day. This'll only take an hour, and then I'll be through."

"What's your housemother like?" Anne asked.

"She's a warden."

"Do you ever see your real mother?"

"Yeah, sometimes."

"How are things between you and her?"

"Fine. I miss her."

"What stops you from being at home with her?"

"I'm under a judge, and I need his approval. My mother has no say."

"Why does he want you here?"

"He's a bastard."

"Why toward you?"

"I come from the wrong side of the tracks. His daughter Lizzy screwed my first boyfriend, right before me and him started going out together. Lizzy's father said to me, 'Why can't you be nice like Lizzy? She don't ever give me problems.' But he doesn't know about her screwing. When I'm seventeen, I'm leaving here."

"What will you do then?"

"I might go to college."

"What will you study?"

"I don't know. Maybe English and writing. I might get married."

"Do you have a boyfriend now?"

"Yeah."

"How long have you been dating him?"

"I can't date him. I've been loving him for a long time, for two years. Sometimes I sneak out and meet him. It's strict here. They won't let you out or let you make a move."

"Maybe they're afraid you'll screw your boyfriend."

"Most of these women don't know what screwing is."

"Do you?" asked Anne.

"What do you think?"

"I don't know."

"Then it's none of your business." Ruth paused. "Do you?" she asked Anne.

"Screw?"

"Yeah."

"I do."

"Believe it or not, I don't," Ruth said.

"Have you had any sexual experience?"

"None."

Anne handed her card VI.

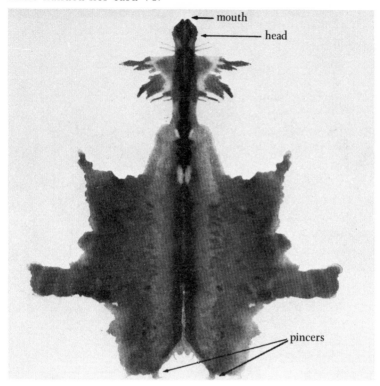

Ruth looked at it. "Some kind of animal with pincers on it."

"Where are the pincers?"

Ruth showed her. "With the head at the other end, the vicious end. There's a mouth on the head."

"Where's the mouth?"

"Here. It's some kind of vicious animal, really."

"It's looking to you a little like a penis, isn't it?" Anne said.

"Yeah. I didn't want you to know I've seen a penis. If you get someone else in here, don't say I said that."

"I wouldn't."

"I'm not worried. They wouldn't believe you anyway."

"You *are* fifteen. It wouldn't be surprising if you'd seen some penises and could recognize the shape of one."

"I've done baby-sitting."

"Do you have a brother? Have you seen his penis?"

"I used to take baths with him, but I don't remember ever having seen it."

"Your boyfriend's penis?"

"I've never seen his."

"What about your father's?"

"No, never. He was very careful never to do that sort of thing." After this trance, when I read back my notes, Ruth said that this was an "absolute lie, because he'd wave it at you when he was drunk."

"It's noteworthy that you put together something vicious and a penis," Anne said. "Why is a penis vicious?"

"You were the one who said it looked like a prick. Why is it vicious to you?"

"It doesn't look vicious to me."

"Does it hurt?"

"What? To screw?"

"Should you be calling it to screw? If we get anyone around here who talks like us, they fire her."

"The main thing is that we both know what we're talking about. No, it doesn't hurt."

"What does it feel like?"

"It doesn't feel like anything else. Are you frightened of it?"

"I've heard that it hurts like hell. Marlene got it when she was thirteen. Something awful happened to her. Her mother sold her for money, so her father brought her here."

"Why did you come here?"

"Everyone who comes here don't come for being screwed. I came because my family wasn't able to take care of me financially. If you don't believe me, read my records."

"Do you believe you were sent here for financial reasons?"

"You sound like all the rest of them. I thought you'd be different. You're not as bad as most, but you could do better."

"How?"

"By not asking so many questions. You can't change anything."

"That's true, though if I had the time, I might be able to help you change the way you feel about the things that have happened."

"Nothing's happened."

"I'm going to have to go," Anne said. "Is there anything you want to ask me before I go?"

"Don't let me keep you."

"Are you angry that I'm going?"

"You come and talk to us, but you couldn't possibly know a hundred and fifty kids. You ask all these nosy questions, but you can't do anything to help. No wonder we're angry at you."

"I haven't seen the other hundred and forty-nine."

"Where are you going?"

"To London."

"Would you take me with you?"

Anne smiled. "Just let me fetch my magic carpet, and we'll be there together in a moment." Anne held Ruth's hand. "O.K., we're going now. You're coming out of it now. And *now* we're in London."

Ruth rubbed her eyes. The trance was over.

"I feel on the verge of crying. I don't know why," Ruth said.

"You were a very difficult adolescent to test," Anne said.

Ruth smiled, and blushed a little.

I noted to myself that during this last trance Anne had told the truth that she did not work for the children's institution, that she was from London, and that Ruth had been "here" since that morning—none of which had seemed to disrupt the trance.

"You reacted differently to Morty in each trance," Anne said. "At seven you didn't pay him any attention; at ten you said at the start that you didn't like him and asked that he move farther away; and at fifteen, you were hostile a few times, with tinges, I thought, of flirting and teasing."

I read aloud my notes of the three trances.

Ruth was surprised that she had given her real name, her baby sister's real name, and Cheepy, her childhood nickname, since in her adult state she had wanted to withhold from Anne identifying information.

Ruth winced upon hearing how she had treated me in the last two trances. "After the rape, I guess I didn't like men," she said, "except for my brother a bit, my uncles, and my boyfriend, whom I adored." She was dismayed at hearing how rude she had been to Anne in the last trance.

"We had a psychologist at the children's home," Ruth said, "who would come in to make sure we were all safe and sane. We'd sit up the night before and decide what symptoms we were going to have. She gave us this word-association test. She couldn't test all of us at one time. Those who'd been tested would tell the others the words, so that they could decide on their responses in advance. Once, after every word I said 'car.' She rapped her pencil on the table and said that if I didn't give answers I'd be punished. I said, 'Well, you said I should say the first thing that comes to mind.' She didn't like the job, and she quit pretty soon after that."

Anne found Ruth fascinating. In a report to me later, Anne wrote, "In all the memory trances, her conversation, style of relating, and responses to the Rorschach cards were convincingly those of a child at corresponding ages, and also accorded with her personal history. Her responses in the same inkblots were very dissimilar to the trances and in her normal state."

Ruth's tears in the trance at ten appeared more like the

response of a ten-year-old than of the adult Ruth. Further, in the trance at fifteen her confusion about being in the room with us instead of at the coast swimming seemed consistent with how she might have behaved had she suddenly found herself in unfamiliar surroundings.

"Admittedly, her performance was impressive," a skeptical voice in my head suggested. "However, she could have been playing a role, encouraged and supported by Anne's expectations, tone, wording, and gestures; your expectations; and her own motivations."

"What you say," replied a trustful voice, "could plausibly explain some of her behavior, but her responses on the inkblot test could have corresponded so closely to a child's of those ages only if she had become a child herself, at least in some sense."

"You can't know that," answered the skeptic, "without having asked her to respond to the test in her normal adult state as she supposed she'd done as a child. You don't know either whether her responses to the inkblots in the memory trances resembled those she'd have given had she actually taken the test at those ages."

I thought these rival arguments had merit, and I could not decide between them. I recognized that I had not anticipated the skeptic's contentions. In Anne's thoughtful and intelligent hands, the Rorschach testing had produced interesting results, but it was a test that was suitable for exploring personality, not for resolving the debate between the skeptical and the trustful voices.

I pondered what had been happening in Ruth's memory trances, since I wanted to understand them better, or at least to clarify my questions about them.

I compared her memory trances to a well-known phenomenon of hypnosis. The hypnotist suggests that the subject return to an earlier period in the subject's life. The subject then displays behavior and has experiences that seem to typify those of the suggested age. The phenomenon is called hypnotic age regression. [25]

It is a striking thing to see a subject regress to the age of a child.

Words and phrases, gestures, emotional responses, handwriting, and drawings may all become childlike, and may conform remarkably closely to those of a child of the suggested age. In hypnotic age regression, the subject's ability to recall occurrences from his or her past may be enhanced. Afterward the subject sometimes has no memory of anything that happened during the hypnosis.

Hypnotic age regressions and Ruth's memory trances seemed similar. The main difference was that Ruth had not been hypnotized—unless her memory trances can be considered a form of self-hypnosis.

There has been much controversy about how to interpret the phenomenon of hypnotic age regression. Can an adult actually return to a child's age? An adult cannot shrink in size. Always, then, it is an adult adopting a child's experience and behavior. Does this mean that the hypnotically regressed person is enacting an adult's conception of what he or she was like at a previous age? Perhaps. However, the person generally does not have any awareness of doing so, during the hypnotic trance or afterward. How closely can the hypnotized adult approximate his or her own experience and behavior as a child? Or approximate the kinds of experience and behavior that characterize most children of that age? The same questions applied to Ruth's memory trances, and I decided to explore them with her.

Whatever the answers to these questions, I thought Ruth's memory trances had given her an unusual opportunity to have psychotherapeutic experiences. Psychotherapists often suppose that someone's adult suffering is an expression of an unhappy child inside, who needs comprehension and help. How much easier their task would be if that child disclosed itself as openly as the child—or children—inside Ruth did! In her memory trances, Ruth had nakedly expressed childhood hurts, and Anne's understanding and sympathy had seemed to benefit her.

Investigating the Memory Trances

RUTH and I were chatting one evening with Vicky Rippere in Vicky's flat. Vicky was a psychologist at the Maudsley Hospital and the Institute of Psychiatry in London, and still is. She had had no experience of hypnotic age regression, but her intellect and scholarship had led me to expect she might have ideas for discovering more about Ruth's memory trances.

Previously, I had told Vicky about Ruth's history, the therapy, the explorations Ruth and I had done, and the memory trances.

"Is there any way of testing," I had asked Vicky, "whether she's putting on a convincing show of a child's behavior or is actually reliving herself as a child?"

Like me, Vicky had been interested in the question out of scientific curiosity. Having been Ruth's therapist, I also hoped that the testing would provide knowledge about Ruth, as the inkblot test had. I expected that her collaborating with a psychologist in research would raise her self-esteem, since all her early contacts with psychologists had been at the children's institution where she had held a status inferior to theirs.

After talking with Vicky and me for about twenty minutes, Ruth began the testing that Vicky had proposed. Ruth found these instructions accompanying the first test:

> On the following page you will find the concept ME and ten pairs of adjectives roughly opposite in meaning. Each pair of adjectives forms a scale. By putting an X in one of the spaces of the scale, you can indicate what you associate with the concept ME, referring to yourself.
>
> The closer you put your X toward either end of the scale, the more strongly you associate ME with the characteristic named. If you don't feel either one way or the other, or equally much like both, then put your X in the middle space. However, it is better not to use the middle space too often.
>
> It is best to work as quickly as you can, without pondering over any scale. Your first impressions are what count.

On the following page, Ruth discovered:

ME

valuable	—:	—:	—:	—:	—:	—:	—	worthless
shallow	—:	—:	—:	—:	—:	—:	—	deep
slow	—:	—:	—:	—:	—:	—:	—	fast
active	—:	—:	—:	—:	—:	—:	—	passive
small	—:	—:	—:	—:	—:	—:	—	large
clean	—:	—:	—:	—:	—:	—:	—	dirty
weak	—:	—:	—:	—:	—:	—:	—	strong
tasty	—:	—:	—:	—:	—:	—:	—	distasteful
relaxed	—:	—:	—:	—:	—:	—:	—	tense
cold	—:	—:	—:	—:	—:	—:	—	hot

This test is known as the Semantic Differential.[26] In cases of multiple personality, psychologists have sometimes been able to distinguish the various individual personalities from each other by administering this test to each personality separately, since each personality may give sharply different responses.

We wanted to see if this test could distinguish Ruth's personalities in memory trances from the person she imagined she had been at corresponding ages.

We also wanted to see if the test could distinguish Ruth in her normal state from the apparition of herself.

Every time Ruth would take this test, the same adjective pairs would be placed in a different order to inhibit any influence upon her answers from a previous testing.

She filled out the Semantic Differential in her normal state, and then turned to the next test, which began with these instructions:

> There are twenty numbered blanks on the following page. Please write twenty answers to the simple question "Who am I?" in the blanks. Just give twenty different answers to this question. Answer as if you were giving the answers to yourself, not to somebody else. Write the answers in the order that they occur to you. Don't worry about logic or "importance." Go along fairly fast, for the time is limited.

This test is called the Twenty Statements Test.[27]

"This is hard," Ruth said, after her first few responses. "I hope I'm giving the right sorts of answers."

"Anything goes," Vicky said.

Ruth wrote some more.

"I hope these answers won't seem silly to you. I'm writing exactly what I feel, O.K.?"

"Silly doesn't come into it," replied Vicky.

Ruth finished. "I think I missed the whole point of it," she said.

Vicky and I had planned that this evening, after Ruth did the Semantic Differential and the Twenty Statements Test in her normal state, she would do them as she imagined she would have at fifteen and as she imagined she would have at ten. On a second evening we would give the same two tests to her apparition, to her in a memory trance at fifteen, and to her in a memory trance at ten. We would then compare her results in her normal state with the apparition's results, her results when she imagined being fifteen with those in a memory trance at fifteen, and her results when she imagined being ten with those in a memory trance at ten.

Ruth filled out her responses to the tests as she imagined she would have at fifteen. "I've done all I can on this," she said, after giving twelve responses on the Twenty Statements Test.

She went on to imagine how she would have done the tests at ten. Again she could give only twelve responses on the Twenty Statements Test. "I answered those just as I think I would have at ten. I'm afraid I've been so honest that you're not going to get anything out of it."

We now told her we would be testing her again, but not that the tests would be the same, or under what conditions she would be taking them, lest she plan her answers.

Vicky and I did not look at Ruth's test responses yet to ensure that we could not use knowledge of them to influence her performance the second time.

When Ruth arrived at Vicky's flat five evenings later, Vicky told her that we would like Ruth's apparition, Ruth in a memory trance at fifteen, and Ruth in a memory trance at ten to take the same tests as before.

"Can I start with the most strenuous first," Ruth asked, "which is me at ten years old?"

Vicky and I agreed.

Ruth closed her eyes and began to enter a memory trance. After about a minute, her eyes opened.

She looked at the instructions for the Semantic Differential and asked me to explain them to her, which I did.

The first pair of adjectives was "cold-hot." "I'm not cold or hot," she said. She put no mark in that first row.

"I don't taste like nothing," she commented after seeing the second pair of adjectives, "tasty" and "distasteful." She did not mark that row either.

In the third row, which was "weak-strong," she put a cross next to "strong."

She looked at the fourth pair of adjectives, "passive-active." "What does 'passive' mean?" she asked me.

"The opposite of active," I said.

"You mean, just not moving?"

"Sort of, but not exactly."

She put a cross in the middle space of that fourth row.

She looked at the fifth pair, "clean-dirty." "I'm not doing it," she said.

"Why not?" I asked.

"None of your business. Besides, it's dumb."

"Just put in an answer."

"Why do you want me to do this?"

"To help me to understand you better."

"Are you some kind of teacher?"

"Sort of."

She looked at the next pair, "deep-shallow." "That's dumb. Can we skip that one?"

"For now."

She read the rest of the adjective pairs. "They're all dumb. You can't make me do any of them."

On the last row she put a cross next to the word "large," which was paired with the word "small." She moved back up the page to the eighth pair, "slow-fast," and put a cross next to "fast." She laid her pencil down. She was finished.

I wanted her to continue. I pointed to the ninth pair, "tense-relaxed." "Are you tense or relaxed?"

"None of your beeswax."

"Could I ask you to do one more?"

"Which one?"

"'Clean-dirty.'"

She picked up her pencil and drew a large circle around the

whole "clean-dirty" row. She started to write something in the upper-right-hand corner of the page. It was her real first name! She followed it with her middle name and maiden name. The handwriting was that of a child, and did not resemble her adult handwriting!

I supposed that by writing her name she was again telling me that she had finished the test.

She put her pencil down.

"Who are you?" she asked. "What's your name?"

"Morty."

"I don't believe you're a teacher."

"I am, sort of."

"I think you're from Welfare."

"I'm not. Try some more of these."

"I told you, I don't want to." Again she picked up her pencil. "I'll make you happy," she said. Starting at the top of the page, she put a cross in the middle space of each of the ten rows without bothering to reread what the adjectives were. "There, I'm through." She put her pencil down.

She took the answer sheet she had just written on, folded it into a paper airplane, and threw it across the room.

"What's next?" she asked.

I gave her the form that had twenty blank numbered spaces and explained what was wanted of her in the Twenty Statements Test.

In the same childlike handwriting, she filled in the first five blank spaces:

[She wrote her real first name]

1 My name is ▓▓▓▓▓

2 I am a girl.

3 I am a Big sister

4 I got one too

5 a school girl

Her writing "I am a 'Big sister'" meant her little sister, Jane, was already alive, which meant, too, her father's assault had occurred.

She wrote her real full name in the upper-right-hand corner of the page. "I'm through," she said. "That's all I can do. Did I do all right? What did I get?"

"There's no grade," I said.

"Then what's it for?"

"To understand you better."

"You're not supposed to do that."

"Why not?"

"You're not my kin. It's none of your business. If you're not really a teacher and you're not from Welfare, and you're not a relative, it's none of your business." She closed her eyes and rested her hand on her forehead. "I feel funny."

"How do you feel funny?"

She gave no answer. She opened her eyes again. "O.K.," she said.

She had come out of the trance on her own.

"Do you remember it?" I asked.

"I can't."

Ruth chose to do the memory trance at fifteen next.

"Where am I?" was the first thing she said upon reaching the trance state.

"You're in a psychologist's apartment."

"A psychologist! Did Miss Finch tell you to do this?"

"No." I recalled in a previous memory trance at fifteen, Ruth had said that her social worker at the children's home had been called Miss Finch.

I handed Ruth the Semantic Differential. She read the instructions and filled it out.

I then gave her the Twenty Statements Test, and she began to write her responses.

As she did, I read quietly from a notebook I had with me.

"I can't do this with you rattling those pages," she said to me.

"I'm sorry. I'll stop." I put the book down.

She resumed writing.

When she finished, she handed the paper to me.

"Thanks," I said.

"You're acting as if I had a choice."

I looked at her responses.

"Are you grading it?" she asked.

"No."

She had responded to the Twenty Statements Test by writing the following:

who am I
1. I am a storm that never arrives
2. I am a dream I haven't dreamed
3. I am a song I'll never sing
4. I am a truth living a lie
5. I am a boat that never comes
6. I am a star that's never shown
7. I am a death that hasn't died
8. I am a trap that has been sprung
9. I am a dream that never ends
10. I am a girl yet I am the wind
11. I am a heart that aches within
12. I am a door I can't get in.
13. I am the wind that's never blown
14. I am a person I've never known
15. I am a tree reaching for you
16. I am a bus going nowhere
17. I am a call you cannot hear
18. I am away
19.   and can't be
20.   near

On the twenty-first and twenty-second lines, she had written "by" and her maiden name.

The handwriting was obviously very different from what it had been in the memory trance at ten; it resembled, but was not the same as, Ruth's adult handwriting.

She picked up a pack of a well-known brand of cigarettes that was lying in front of her on Vicky's desk. "My momma smokes these and hides them," she said.

"Why does she hide them?" I asked.

"Any lady wouldn't be caught out in public smoking these. Don't you know that, darling?" She said it slowly, with her little finger up in the air, and with the affectation of an upper-class, middle-aged American socialite. "Have you got a match?"

I offered her one.

"I smoke these all the time," she said, as I lit her cigarette.

She started to cough after taking two puffs. It was the cough of a novice smoker.

"They're not my brand," she said.

"What is your brand?" I asked.

"I prefer mentholated cigarettes. That cigarette didn't choke me. I just had something in my throat."

She saw me taking notes on what she was saying. "I didn't tell you you could do that," she said.

"I hadn't realized I needed your permission." I went on writing.

"I'm going to tell Miss Finch what you're doing. She's the only one who can know about me. What are you doing this for anyway?"

"For you," I answered.

"You can't adopt me. I'm too old."

By "for you," I had meant for her benefit. She had understood "for you" to mean for the sake of obtaining her. Her misunderstanding was perhaps related to her having spent many years at a children's home.

"I didn't mean I wanted to adopt you."

"Can I go?" she asked.

"Yes," I replied.

"Who's picking me up?"

"Who usually does?"

"I don't know how I got here." She paused for a moment. "That would be a joke," she said.

"What would?"

"Amnesia." She laughed.

"Amnesia for what?"

"Isn't that what you call it when you forget?"

"Yes."

"Who are you?"

"I'm a psychiatrist."

"Oh, God!" She tapped her pencil on the table in annoyance. "I guess you know all shrinks are nuts."

"Oh?"

"They must be nuts. Otherwise why would they want to be with crazy people all the time? Can I go now?"

"Yes."

"Can I have my paper back?" She tried to grab it from my hands.

"No," I said, pulling it away from her.

"You're a real shitass."

She turned her face away suddenly, closed her eyes, opened them again, and then looked at me. She was out of the trance.

"I'm trembling all over," she said. "I'd like to stop for coffee."

After a few minutes' chat, Vicky told Ruth that we would like Ruth's apparition to fill out the same two tests.

"This time I won't be in a trance," Ruth said, "so I'll remember what happens."

Ruth pointed to my chair, which was next to hers. "I'll put the apparition there."

I changed chairs.

"Isn't he courteous to my apparition?" she said to Vicky.

Ruth and her apparition looked at the Semantic Differential together. The apparition dictated to her the answers, and Ruth wrote them down.

Ruth finished the test. "My apparition and I had a few disagreements there, but I put down what she said. O.K.?"

"O.K.," I replied.

After filling out eight statements on the Twenty Statements Test, Ruth said, "I can't hold her here any longer."

"Try to bring her back if you can," I said, "for some more statements."

She did. She filled out two more statements, making ten altogether, and then stopped.

Now that the tests were over, we told Ruth why we had tested her. By comparing her test results in her normal state of mind with those of her apparition, we hoped to determine whether the apparition had a personality distinct from Ruth or was a representation of Ruth's own personality.[28]

"I'm absolutely positive that the apparition of me is part of myself," was Ruth's reaction.

If the apparition was a part of Ruth, it still had a special awareness, as it had told her things about herself that she had not been consciously aware of knowing, and had also given her a method for recalling events that she had seemingly not thought of before.

We now took our first look at Ruth's test results in her normal state. On the Semantic Differential, she had marked the spaces nearest to "tasty," "clean," "deep," and "valuable"—and, we found, so had the apparition. Ruth and the apparition had only three times given answers that differed by more than one space. The apparition had marked the space nearest to "slow," whereas Ruth had marked the space five spaces nearer to "fast." Perhaps the difference was related to the apparition's having answered the test more slowly than Ruth had. The apparition had put a cross midway between "hot" and "cold," whereas Ruth had marked the space nearest to "hot." Perhaps the apparition—or Ruth—knew that apparitions are supposed to feel cooler to the touch than live persons. The apparition had marked the space nearest to "strong," while Ruth had put a cross midway between strong and weak.

Generally, Ruth's and the apparition's responses resembled each other more than the responses given by two separate people or by two distinct personalities within the same person.[29]

On the Twenty Statements Test, Ruth had written:

1. I am me.
2. I am alone sometimes.
3. I am good.
4. I am happy.
5. I am hurt.
6. I am smart but not educated.

7. I am sincere.
8. I am a person of sensitive feelings.
9. I am a part of all that is.
10. I am brave.
11. I am a coward.
12. I am a queen.
13. I am a pauper.
14. I am a friend.
15. I am confused.
16. I am excited.
17. I am trying.
18. I am feeling.
19. I am lost but not afraid of being lost.
20. I am *thru!*

On the same test, the apparition had made only ten statements. Its first response was "I am you," which seemed to parody Ruth's first response, made five days earlier, "I am me," and which also seemed to say that the apparition *was* Ruth, not a personality distinct from Ruth. Confirming this interpretation was the apparition's second response, "We are one." Its third response was "I am the queen of Persia," which is related to Ruth's response, "I am a queen." Its fourth and fifth responses were "I am the mother of three" and "I am a wife." Both are true of Ruth; they would apply to the apparition if it had its own three children and husband—which we had not heard about—or if it and Ruth were the same person. Its sixth response was "I am a being." Its seventh was "I am a spirit," which was its only statement that seemed to apply to it and not to Ruth and that also distinguished it from Ruth. Its eighth response was "I am sincere," which was identical with Ruth's seventh response. Its ninth response was "I am the best at what I do." Its last statement, "I am tired," was a comment about the present situation, as was Ruth's last statement, "I am *thru!*"

Ruth's responses in her normal state and her apparition's responses on the Semantic Differential and the Twenty Statements Test were compatible with Ruth's assertion that the apparition was part of herself.

We now turned to the Semantic Differential in the "imagine" and trance conditions. In all four trance responses at ten, Ruth had made marks nearest to one end of a row. These responses are consistent with those of a child, as children tend to give extreme ratings on the Semantic Differential, a fact which Ruth had no way of knowing, as far as I could tell. By contrast, in the "imagine" condition at ten, she had placed eight of the ten crosses in either the middle space or the space next to the middle one.

In her trance responses at fifteen, she had again preferred extreme ratings, marking the space at the end of a row eight times; she had done this only twice in the "imagine" condition at fifteen.[30]

She had marked the space nearest "strong" in both trances and the space nearest "weak" in both "imagine" conditions. She had put a cross nearest "tasty" in the trance at fifteen—and over the cross had written the word "very," whereas she had marked the space one space away from "distasteful" when she had imagined being fifteen. At both ages, she had consistently rated herself more favorably in the trances than in the "imagine" conditions.

The answers in the memory trances were as different from those in the "imagine" conditions as if they had been given by different personalities.

On her Twenty Statements Test at ten: in the "imagine" condition she had used her adult handwriting, but in the trance's a child's. In the "imagine" condition she had spelled and capitalized words correctly, but in the trance had written "gilr" and "I am a Big sister." In the "imagine" condition her first response had been "I am my name," but in the trance it had been "My name is ———" and she had written her real name. Writing her real name, which she had done three times in the trance at ten, was consistent with her reliving herself at ten, since at ten she would not have hesitated to give her name, whereas she, the adult, wanted to conceal her identity from Vicky. Writing her maiden name was also compatible with her reliving herself at ten.

When imagining being fifteen, she had given twelve statements on the Twenty Statements Test, none of which were metaphorical, unlike all her statements in the trance at fifteen. Except for "I am hate" and "I am what I am," the statements in the "imagine" condition at fifteen were prosaic and banal, whereas the trance statements at fifteen had been quite the contrary. Some of her responses when imagining being fifteen seemed to reflect ordinary adolescent preoccupations—"I am shy," "I am in love," "I am alone," whereas none of the trance responses at fifteen can be considered ordinary. In the "imagine" condition she had stated "I am a girl," whereas in the trance she had written "I am a girl yet I am the wind," which seems to typify the difference between the two sets of responses at fifteen.

The Twenty Statements Test results suggested that in the memory trances at ten and fifteen, Ruth had had a very different personality than she had imagined she had had at those ages.

In summary: Ruth in her normal state and the apparition of Ruth gave responses on both tests that were so similar as to suggest they came from the same personality. In a memory trance at ten and in imagining herself at ten, the responses on both tests were so different from each other as to suggest they came from different personalities. And the same was so in the trance and "imagine" conditions at fifteen. In the trances her responses on both tests were consistent with those of an actual girl at the corresponding ages.

"Your behavior in the memory trances seemed so authentic," Vicky said to Ruth, "that if the test results had been different than they were, I'd have supposed something was wrong with the tests."

After hearing what had happened in the trances, Ruth said, "I don't remember any of that. I wish I could."

"Why don't you write a note to yourself about your feelings while you're still in a trance?" Vicky said. "You could then refer to it afterward."

"I don't know if I could remember to do that in a trance," Ruth replied.

I drove Ruth to the place where she was staying the night.

"I think the trance at ten was after the rape," she said, "and that ten-year-old didn't want to answer about 'clean' and 'dirty,' because she believed you were insulting her and supposed she was dirty."

"I agree," I said.

"She was defying you," Ruth said. "I sounded a lot more disturbed at ten than at fifteen. At fifteen, it seems I'd built up an immunity, an 'I don't care' attitude. Do you think you'd have liked that ten- and fifteen-year-old? Would you have wanted to get to know them better?"

"I might have liked them if they'd have given me a chance to. But I doubt they'd have let me get to know them."

"Do you think they needed to see a psychiatrist?"

"I don't think they would have wanted to. They had too much to hide."

The next morning Vicky phoned me.

"Would you like to know how she compares with the Ruth you'd described?" Vicky said. "My personal reaction, I mean."

"Yes?"

"She's more playful, friendly, and outgoing than I'd expected and has a good sense of humor. Besides being fascinating, she's a lot of fun."

"There's something bothering me," I said. "How do we know that she didn't consciously and deliberately imagine herself at younger ages in both the 'imagine' and trance conditions, and did so halfheartedly in the 'imagine' conditions and wholeheartedly in the trances?"

"We don't know," Vicky said, "since we can't know what was going on in her mind. But her performance in the trances was so realistic. To have acted as well as she did, she'd have had to rehearse it. How vividly does one have to imagine before 'imagine' passes over into being an age regression or a memory trance?"

Unexpectedly, I came upon another method for exploring

whether Ruth was reliving herself as a young girl in the memory trances.

She once told me she had had a photographic memory as a child: "My first reading book, when I was in the second grade, had about twenty words on a page. I read it first by myself and then to my mother, who wanted to hear me read. I'd read a page to her, and before she'd turn the page, I'd recite the next one to her.

"There's a card game called Concentration. All the cards are laid facedown and spread out. Two cards at a time are turned over, so the players can see the cards' faces, and then are turned facedown again. The game tests the players' skills at remembering the faces of the cards, and the one who has the best memory usually wins. As a child, I used to beat every kid on the block.

"Because of my memory, my parents thought I should do well in school. Yet I didn't. I didn't pay attention in class, and books bored me. I was terrified whenever I got a good grade, because if it later fell, my parents would spank me or restrict me to the house until the next report card.

"My mother told people I had a photographic memory, but didn't use it. My ability just made my life difficult. It was something to be bitched at about. So I decided to lose it. I doubt I still have it."

Some children can stare at an image, such as a picture, for a minute or less and maintain it before their eyes, after the image has been removed. The image they recreate is remarkably clear and detailed, and is at times surprisingly faithful to the original image. It can be vivid enough to blot out the background against which it is projected. The child can "turn on" the image voluntarily, sometimes weeks after having first been exposed to it, and can keep it stationary in space to scan it. The images these children form are called "eidetic images," and the children are called "eidetikers."[31] The ability to produce eidetic images is common in children—estimates of its incidence vary from 8 to 60 percent—but rare after eleven years old.

Ruth's remarks about her "photographic memory" suggested that she had been an "eidetiker." I wondered if her ability to create apparitions might be related to a talent for eidetic imagery. Was she still an "eidetiker" or had she lost the talent, as she believed?

Ruth and I, at the Brain and Perception Laboratory of the University of Bristol, with John Harris, a research psychologist, and Richard L. Gregory, the professor, stared at a picture showing the heads and shoulders of five men, each wearing a different top, two wearing glasses, three wearing hats of different kinds, and one bald. A series of nine random letters that did not form a word appeared above each man's head, and six numbers appeared below each man. The picture, called the Rogues' Gallery, was devised to test an ability for eidetic imagery.

After a minute, John removed the picture and asked Ruth what she saw now on the blank white paper upon which the picture had been resting.

She told us. She was correct about many features of the picture and though she made mistakes, especially with the letters and numbers, she did better than most adults could.

Was she an "eidetiker"? That she had made mistakes did not necessarily mean she was not, since eidetic imagery generally involves some inaccuracies. The results were inconclusive.

It now occurred to me to see whether she could recover in a memory trance the "photographic memory" of her childhood. If she could, it would strengthen the view that she was reliving herself as a child in the trances.

I tested her ability again in her normal adult state, this time with Max Coltheart present. Max is professor of psychology at London University's Birkbeck College and has done research with visual imagery.

I gave Max a handful of my children's illustrated books and suggested he choose a picture from one of them.

Ruth stared for a minute at the picture he had chosen, before I removed it. In response to questions from Max and me, she described the picture's details.

Her performance was much better than with the picture of the Rogues' Gallery. Perhaps that first time had been practice for her, perhaps this time she was trying harder or perhaps she was better with people and objects than with letters and numbers.

"I've been looking for an adult eidetiker for ten years," Max said, "and you're the first one I've met."

"What good does it do me?" Ruth asked. "You don't get a degree for it, do you? And it can't make me money!"

"Aren't you pleased that you're educating Max and me?" I said.

"Big deal!" she replied.

I asked her to return in a memory trance to seven years old and try with another picture. Seven was the age at which she thought her "photographic memory" had been strongest.

Max chose another picture from the same book.

This time she performed much better than she just had in her normal state. It was obvious to Max and me that, after the picture was removed, she retained the image of it in front of her eyes much longer in her memory trances than she had in her normal state.

I played the same game with her twice more, each time with different pictures, which she had not previously seen. All the pictures were the same size, with approximately the same amount of detail, from the same children's book, and by the same artist.

In her normal state, she kept the image of the picture in front of her eyes the first time for fifty-seven seconds before it faded, and the second time for sixty-seven seconds. In a memory trance at seven years old, she did it the first time for four minutes and fifty-five seconds and the second time for five minutes and thirty seconds. She was apparently a much better eidetiker in a memory trance at seven than in her normal adult state.

The second time we tried it in a memory trance, I handed her the picture of Old Blind Mole from that children's book.[32] The picture showed a mole standing upright and dressed like a gentleman, an insect standing upright and smoking a pipe, and some strawberries and flowers.

"Why don't you look at this picture all over," I said. "Try and look at it carefully, so that you'll remember it afterward."

"O.K. What animal is that?"

"A mole."

"What's a mole?"

"It's like a rat."

"It does look kind of like a rat."

She stared at it for a minute, before I took it away and substituted a blank piece of white paper. "Could you look at that and tell me what you see?" I said.

"I see the mole, and I see a bug, and I see some clouds, and I see some strawberries, and I see everything."

"How many strawberries do you see?"

She stared at the paper for a few seconds. "Ten," she said.

There were ten.

"What color are the clouds?"

"Blue and pink."

She was right.

"Do you see any flowers?" I asked.

"Yes."

"Tell me about them."

"They're white with yellow middles."

Again she was right.

"Can you count them?"

"Three."

There were three.

"Now if you look at the mole, what's it wearing on its head?"

"A hat."

She was correct.

"And can you tell me anything about that hat?"

"It's got a pin in it."

It had a pin.

". . . and it's two different colors."

In fact, it was two very different shades of gray.

"Do you see anything beside the pin on it?"

"Yes. A piece of ribbon."

The hat had a band around it.

"Can you tell me anything about the mole's face?"

"He looks like a rat."

"Yes, he does. What color is his face?"

"Black and pink."

That was correct.

"Do you see his mouth?"

"A little bit."

"What's it like?"

"It's kind of opened."

It was.

"Any teeth?"

"I don't see any. No, he's got some. His shirt's too long for his coat. It's sticking out of his sleeves."

She was right about the presence of the teeth and the shirt.

"What color is his shirt?"

"White."

It was.

"Tell me about the mole's hands."

"They're pink."

They were.

"And he's got a ring on."

"Can you see which finger the ring is on?"

"It's on this one." She held up the first finger of her right hand.

In fact, the mole was holding a cane by means of a strap that went around that finger.

"He's holding the stick," she said.

"That's right. Can you tell me anything about that stick?"

"It's got a silver top and it's a brown stick."

That was correct.

"It's a walking stick."

"Right. And what color is the mole's coat?"

"Dark blue."

It was dark blue.

"Tell me about the mole's pocket."

"It's got worms in it."

"How many worms do you see?"

"Six pink worms."

There were six pink worms.

"Are there any buttons on the mole's coat?"

"He's got one on the sleeve and one at the back, but you can't see the one at the back too good."

She was right.

"O.K. What do you see by the mole's feet?"

"I see some black socks with buttons."

His spats were white.

"The mole's got funny shoes. Why are his toes sticking out?"

"I don't know."

His toes were protruding.

"What do you see in the lower-right-hand corner?" I asked.

"I see a bug. He's got red backs and a hat on."

The insect's red back was divided down the middle into two segments, and he wore a hat.

"Does the bug have anything in its hands?" I asked.

"It's got a pipe."

It did.

"It's got something else," she said.

"What's that?"

"I don't know."

It was holding a walking stick.

"Tell me about the bug's hat."

"It's a magic man's hat."

"Can you describe it?"

"It's black."

It was tan.

"Does it have a band?"

"Yes."

"What color?"

"A bright one."

It was two tones: bright pink above and pale violet below.

"What about the bug's feet?"

"It's got shoes on."

It did.

"What color are they?"

"I think they're yellow."

Its toenails were yellow.

"It's getting hard for me to see it."

The image had faded, but the memory trance continued.

"I want to ask you a different kind of question," I said. "Can you tell me who the president of the United States is?" I wanted to see if she would name the man who had been president when she had been seven.

She looked at me silently.

"You don't know?" I asked.

"Do you still like me?"

"Of course I still like you."

"There's going to be a new one," she said.

"Do you know when?"

"Maybe next year. There's one man somewhere."

"Yes?"

"He might be the president."

"What's his name?"

"Ike. That's a funny name," she said.

"Yes, it is."

I calculated from the date of birth that she had been seven in 1959, the last year of Eisenhower's presidency; in 1960, Kennedy had been elected.

"Do you want me to show you something?" she asked.

"Yes."

"Do you know how to make a bald-headed golfer?"

"No."

"It's a trick."

"All right."

"You got to do it."

"O.K."

She drew three parallel lines on a piece of paper.

"You make a bald-headed golfer," she said.

"What do I do?"

"You make a bald-headed golfer."
"I don't know how."
"You want me to show you?"
"Yes."
She drew:

I EK

"That's a very good trick," I said. "It fooled me. How did you know Ike is a bald-headed golfer?"
"Someone at school showed this to me."
"Is that the right way to spell 'Ike'?"
She looked at the paper. "That's how the girl who showed me spelled it."
"Before we stop for today, I have something to tell you. When you're grown up, I want you to remember this meeting and what happened in it."
"You're not playing with me no more?"
"No. I'm going to leave you now, but I want you to make sure you remember this day and this meeting with me when you grow up. O.K.?"
"That's easy."
"Good. You can grow up now. You can come back now."
A moment passed.
She smiled. "I remember it this time!" she exclaimed.
I asked her about what had just been occurring, and her recall seemed as good as for any nontrance experience she might have just been having.
I did not know why she had previously been amnesic for the trances' contents or why my suggestion succeeded. Similarly, hypnotists do not understand why age-regressed subjects sometimes cannot remember their trances afterward or why the

hypnotist's telling the subject during the trance to remember it afterward can help the subject to do so.

What did it mean that Ruth was a better eidetiker in memory trances at seven than in her normal state? Perhaps she had tried harder to do well in the trances. Perhaps just being in a trance had somehow improved her ability. Or had she truly recovered in the trances a forgotten talent? As I had not seen her actually perform at seven, and as no objective record of her childhood skill exists, I could not compare her skill then with her trance skill.

However her capabilities as an eidetiker in the trances are interpreted, they seemed remarkable.

"Do you have other ideas," I asked Max, "for testing whether in her memory trances she behaves like a real child or like an adult playing the part of a child?"

Max looked thoughtful for a moment. "Bring her along to my lab," he said, "and we'll see."

In Max's laboratory, Ruth returned in a memory trance to three years old and looked through a viewer at some cards that Nick Stirling was flashing at her, one at a time. Nick, a graduate student in Max Coltheart's psychology department, had done research with the test he was now giving Ruth.[33] Each card had a row of four Xs; on some cards all four Xs were colored red, on some green, and on some blue. As soon as Ruth saw the card, she called out the color. A microphone in front of her mouth was attached to a machine that measured precisely how much time elapsed between Nick's inserting the card in the viewer and her uttering a sound. If she said, "Uh, red," the machine measured the time until "Uh." Her naming the colors of the Xs was practice for the real test, which came next.

On each card of this next group was the word RED, GREEN, or BLUE, which was written in either red, green, or blue ink. The word and the ink's color sometimes agreed and sometimes disagreed. Ruth had to name the ink's color as soon as she saw the card.

On this test, a person takes longer to name the ink's color when it and the word disagree than when they agree; the delay in the "disagree" condition, called the interference effect, occurs unless the person cannot read the word—as would be the case with a child who has not learned to read yet.

I had chosen three years old for Ruth's memory trance because she had once told me she had begun learning to read at about five or six.

I had not explained to her the purpose of the testing, lest she try to influence its results. I had simply asked her to return to three, saying I would tell her why later.

Nick presented thirty-six cards in random order; on eighteen cards the word agreed with the ink's color, and on eighteen it did not.

After giving her responses and emerging from the trance, Ruth told me she had gone back to a time in her first months at the children's home.

I asked Ruth to enter a memory trance at seven. I had chosen seven, because I believed she could read by that age and would show the interference effect when the word and the ink's color disagreed.

"Are you a doctor?" she asked me when the trance had begun.

"Yes," I said.

"Will I get a shot?"

"No," I replied.

Nick played the same game with her as before, starting with her looking at the Xs for practice and naming their colors.

In the next group of cards, when she saw the word BLUE written in red ink, she said, "That's a red-blue"; when she saw RED written in green, she said, "That's a green-red"; and when she saw GREEN written in green, she said, "That's a green-green." Her thumb was in her mouth through most of this testing.

When the test was over, Nick left the room briefly.

"You know what?" Ruth said. "That man don't know his colors. He missed a lot of them. Is that man a teacher?"

"Sort of," I said.

I signaled her to come out of the trance, and she did.

"The room just jumped," she said. "I feel dizzy."

Nick returned to the room and, using the same procedure once more, tested her in her normal adult state.

At my request, Nick had left the room just before and just after each of the three testings so that he had not seen her enter or emerge from the trances. He had not been told why she was being tested, and I had not wanted him to know which three states she was in lest he somehow unwittingly influence the results.

I now told him what three states she had been in. He had guessed that once or twice she might have been in a trance, he said, but had not recognized that she had been age regressed.

After I explained to Ruth the point of the testing, she, Max, Nick, and I looked at the results. We found that when the word and the color of the ink had disagreed, she had exhibited the expected delayed response in her normal adult state, but not in either trance. Instead, in the trances, especially in the one at seven, she had responded *more* quickly in the "disagree" than in the "agree" condition.[34]

In the trance at seven, she had read the names of the colors. Why then had she displayed no interference effect in the "disagree" condition?

"A child whose reading is weak," Max said, "reads the word too slowly for it to interfere with the response to the ink's color. Research has discovered that many seven-year-old children don't show an interference effect for this reason."[35]

Perhaps in the trance at seven she had been reliving herself as a child whose reading was weak. In that trance she might have sometimes said "That's a red-blue," "That's a green-red," and so on, because she was having trouble reading the words and was giving herself time. This could have affected the result, since the machine measured the time until she said "That's."

The outcome of the experiment can be interpreted as supporting the possibility that in the memory trances Ruth was reliving herself as a child. The absence of an interference effect in her trance at seven strengthens this interpretation, especially as I had mistakenly supposed that all children who can read show it, and that therefore she would in that trance.[36]

What conclusions did the research into Ruth's memory trances suggest? All the results indicated that in the trances she was somehow different from her usual, normal self. Was she reliving herself as a child in the trances? All the facts—except one—fitted this explanation. The exception was that, unlike an actual child, she could become an adult upon a signal from another person.

Could the results be otherwise explained? A subject who is asked to feign a child's behavior can sometimes closely imitate the phenomenon of hypnotic age regression, especially if another person is present who expects the subject to become a child and treats the subject accordingly. Could Ruth have been playing a game and pretending to be a child? She gave me no reason to suspect her of this. On the last test, she would have had to have guessed its purpose, that children who cannot read show no interference effect, and that children who cannot read well also do not, a fact which I had not realized and which Ruth was most unlikely to have been aware of. She would also have had to have decided to concoct the results she displayed, somehow controlled her trance responses in the "disagree" condition so as to show no interference effect, and controlled all her responses so as not to arouse Nick's mistrust—a very difficult feat when measurements are being made in thousandths of seconds.

An Unusual Brain

A S the reader knows, I had never experienced any of the apparitions that Ruth allegedly experienced. A debate between my skeptical and trustful voices was still unresolved: was there a way of verifying her apparitional experiences?

I asked Peter B. C. Fenwick this question after telling him about Ruth. Peter is a psychiatrist and neurophysiologist who works in London at the Institute of Psychiatry and at St. Thomas' Hospital. He was fascinated with her story. He was eager to meet her and learn more about her avowed ability.

Peter's response pleased me. An important reason for Ruth's improved mental state, I believed, was that she now saw her unusual experiences as evidence of a talent instead of as symptoms of craziness. I expected that Peter's expression of interest in her talent would strengthen her view of herself as talented.

One idea Peter had for testing whether her alleged hallucinations were genuine involved a method that can be used to diagnose hysterical blindness and deafness. Suppose a person says that he or she cannot see, and despite a thorough search by the doctor, no physical cause is found. The doctor suspects the person is suffering from hysterical blindness, meaning the person is imitating, though not consciously, the condition of being blind. It is sometimes difficult to corroborate the presence of hysteria, but in recent years doctors have been helped by a test based on measuring brain waves.

If one repeatedly flashes a bright light at a normal person's eyes, the light will evoke electrical waves from the part of the brain concerned with vision. These waves, which indicate that the brain is responding to the flash, are called the visual evoked response. Someone who is blind from a physical cause does not display a normal visual evoked response, whereas someone who is hysterically blind usually does. The hysteric reports no awareness of the light, but his or her brain responds to it, which signifies that the hysteric's visual mechanisms are functioning normally.

Similarly, a doctor can distinguish deafness of physical origin from hysterical deafness by delivering clicks to the ears and measuring the auditory evoked responses, thereby determining whether the parts of the brain that deal with hearing are responding normally to the clicks.[37]

Peter suggested flashing a light at Ruth and asking her to produce an apparition between the light and her eyes. She had alleged that apparitions blocked objects behind them; this indicated that the apparition might interfere with her experiencing the light, but what would her visual evoked response show? Would the apparition inhibit it, as a real person or object would, or would her brain continue to respond to the light? Then we might go on to test whether an apparition could somehow interfere with her brain's response to clicks. While awaiting the start of the experiment, I remembered how a teacher had once explained the visual and auditory evoked responses to me.

Electrodes on the scalp can detect the brain's electrical activity, and the tracing of that activity on paper is called the electroencephalogram (EEG). Looking at an EEG tracing is rather like listening to the sounds of a large city from a position several miles above it. You could tell from the noise roughly how busy or awake the city's occupants were, but not what any particular individuals were doing. Now imagine that the city has a large sports stadium in which thousands of people are sitting. Imagine that we can provoke them to roar full-throatedly in unison exactly one second after they see a light flashed at them. From our position above the city, the roar is undetectable, as it is drowned out by the other city noises. If we flashed the light at precisely one-minute intervals, recorded all the noise over fifteen or twenty minutes, divided our recording into one-minute segments such that each segment began at the moment the light flashed, and used a computer to sample at hundreds of moments the noise on each segment and to add up and average the samples, we would retrieve the sound of the roars. That is because the noise from the rest of the city varies somewhat randomly, being loud one moment and soft the next, while the crowd's roars occur at exactly the same moment in each one-minute interval. The crowd's roar is comparable to the response evoked by a flash or click from the brain areas concerned with vision or hearing, and the random city noises are comparable to the electrical activity of the brain as a whole. Because the brain's general activity masks the evoked responses, a series of them must be produced and added together by a computer before they become detectable.

Ruth sat in Peter's laboratory looking at a flashing lamp two feet in front of her eyes. Behind her, her brain's electical activity was being displayed on a screen called an oscilloscope.

"How's my brain working?" Ruth asked Peter.

"You've got a good visual evoked response," Peter replied.

"I understood the word 'good,' but that's all."

Peter laughed. "Your brain is working fine. Could you make an apparition between yourself and the lamp?"

"I'll try. I'll raise my finger to let you know when I'm seeing one." She stared at the lamp. After about a minute she raised a finger, and Peter immediately turned the computer on. After sixteen flashes she lowered her finger, indicating the apparition was no longer there.

The oscilloscope showed Ruth's visual evoked response during the time the apparition was allegedly present was about half the intensity it had previously been.

"What did you experience?" I asked Ruth.

"I made an apparition of my daughter, Heather, sitting on my lap, so that her head was in front of my eyes. I saw her little head facing the lamp, the part in her hair, and her pigtails. She blocked out the lamp, but I could still see light around her head. It was like before a sunrise or after a sunset when the sun is below the horizon, and the sky near the sun is golden."

"How do you make an apparition?" asked Peter.

"I stop paying attention to everything around me. I decide whose apparition I want to make. I remember what the person looks like, as most people might with their eyes closed—except my eyes are open. And I produce the person."

"Let's try again," I said, "and this time, to eliminate the corona of light, why don't you have Heather face you, and put her hands on your eyes?"

"All right."

Ruth tried what I suggested, keeping her eyes open. The result was a visual evoked response of about the same intensity as when Heather had faced the lamp.

We measured Ruth's visual evoked response two more times without her making an apparition—once with Ruth's eyes covered with my hands, which were presumably bigger than Heather's apparitional ones, and once with Ruth's eyes closed. Each time the visual evoked response was about as intense as when Heather's apparition had been there, and about half as intense as when Ruth had first looked at the lamp, with her eyes open and no apparition there.

How were we to understand the results? The apparition had seemed to inhibit Ruth's visual evoked response, but had not eliminated it. The other maneuvers we had tried had had a similar effect. Peter guessed the response Ruth was showing represented an auditory evoked response, since the lamp had made a noise whenever it had flashed, and the response thereby evoked from the auditory parts of Ruth's brain could have been transmitted to our recording electrodes.

Peter now asked Ruth to stare at a television screen that displayed a checkerboard pattern in which the white squares repetitively changed to black ones and the black ones to white ones at a rate of about once a second. This is another means of eliciting a visual evoked response. The checkerboard squares changed color noiselessly, so that there would be no auditory evoked response.

Ruth's visual evoked response to the checkerboard pattern reversals was normal.

She again produced an apparition of Heather sitting on her lap to block her experience of the screen.

The electrical activity of Ruth's brain during sixteen pattern reversals was averaged. Her visual evoked response was completely absent!

"You've won!" Peter exclaimed.

"What's happened?" Ruth asked.

"Your brain has behaved in the same way it would have if your daughter had actually been sitting on your lap," Peter said. "You've produced the appearance of a real person."

"But I could have told you that," Ruth replied.

"Yes, but your saying so isn't the same as our proving it."

We repeated the experiment several times. When Ruth said her daughter's head blocked the checkerboard pattern incompletely, the visual evoked response was reduced but not eliminated. Ruth's reports of how completely the screen in front of her was obstructed consistently corresponded with how much the visual evoked response displayed on the oscilloscope behind her was inhibited.

"It's nice that you can tell us what's going on with the electrodes," Peter said.

"It's nice that the electrodes can tell you what I'm seeing," she replied.

Peter wanted to ensure that the elimination of her visual evoked response had been due to the apparition and nothing else. While she stared at the apparition blocking the screen, he looked at her pupils to see if they were converging, since convergence of the pupils throws the pattern out of focus and can reduce the visual evoked response. The pupils, he found, were not converging.

While she continued to face the screen, he asked her to converge her pupils deliberately, without producing an apparition. She did, and her visual evoked response diminished, but remained prominent.

He asked her to stare at the screen and to imagine, but not hallucinate, her daughter on her lap, since paying attention to something other than the pattern reversals can in itself reduce the visual evoked response. When she did, her evoked response diminished, but not as much as when she had hallucinated her daughter.

He suggested she subtract serial sevens from one hundred while staring at the screen, and the same result occurred.

Once again he called upon her to block out the screen fully by means of an apparition sitting on her lap. She did, and the evoked response disappeared altogether.

"I'm convinced," said Peter.

"Is my brain functioning all right?" asked Ruth.

"Your brain can do things that mine and Morty's can't. Want to trade?"

Later, Peter told the results to a psychiatrist colleague. The psychiatrist asked if Ruth's eyes had been open. Peter said they had. The psychiatrist asked if Peter was sure that Ruth had not painted pictures of her eyes on her eyelids beforehand, so that she would seem to have her eyes open when they were shut.

As that conversation suggests, our results were most unusual.

Where did Ruth's brain intercept the visual stimuli that she stopped seeing when the apparitions got in the way?

Was her retina, the light-sensitive surface at the back of her eye, registering the stimuli?

In the laboratory of Dr. Hisako Ikeda, head of the Vision Research Unit at London's St. Thomas' Hospital, an electroretinogram, which measures the retina's electrical response to light, showed that Ruth's retina responded normally to a beam of light shining at her eye.

Ruth now had Paul's apparition shield her eye from the light with its hand. The recording apparatus on her eye prevented Paul's hand from covering her eye completely, and she reported still seeing some light but less light than before the hand was there.

The electroretinogram showed no change.

We turned the light off, and in complete darkness, Ruth had Paul's apparition turn the light on. She reported seeing some light, though less than when the light had actually been on.

The electroretinogram again showed no change.

That the apparition had not affected the responses of her retina was unsurprising, as retinal responses are not controlled by the brain's cerebral cortex, where consciousness and will originate. We now knew that the blocking of her visual evoked response to light had occurred after the light had been normally registered by her retina.

Would her pupils constrict in response to a hallucinatory light beam? Dilate in response to the hallucinatory obstruction of an actual light beam?

Doctors Stephen E. Smith and Christopher J. K. Ellis of St. Thomas' Hospital and I tested this with a sophisticated instrument for measuring pupillary diameter called a scanning pupillometer, which displays enlarged images of the pupils on a television screen.

The results were that her pupils responded normally to actual light and actual darkness, but were unaffected by the apparition's turning the light on or off, except for showing the slight dilation that normally accompanies concentrating on a task.

This meant that the blocking of her visual evoked response had occurred by pathways to the brain other than those controlling the pupils' adaptation to darkness and light.

* * *

Back in Peter's laboratory, Ruth sat with earphones listening to clicks being delivered at a rate of about two a second.

Peter measured her auditory evoked response and found it to be normal.

"Could you have your daughter put her hands over your ears, so you don't hear the clicks?" Peter said.

"The earphones would fall off if she tried to get her hands right on my ears," Ruth replied. "I'll try and get her to take the earphones from my ears and put them elsewhere in the room."

Ruth did. "I can still vaguely hear the clicks," she said. The oscilloscope behind her confirmed her remark, as it showed her auditory evoked response was diminished, but still present.

"Could your daughter turn down the volume control on the machine producing the clicks to the point where you can't hear them?" Peter said, and he showed Ruth the control knob.

"Could I try it with the lights out?" Ruth asked. "When you and Morty look at me while I do it, I feel self-conscious and can't concentrate."

We turned out the lights.

When Ruth signaled to us with her finger that her daughter was turning down the volume, Peter put on the computer.

The electrical activity of Ruth's brain during thirty-two clicks was averaged. Her auditory evoked response was completely absent! [38]

"That's a winner!" said Peter.

"I knew I'd done it that time," said Ruth. "As a child at school, I used to turn off the teacher's voice so that when she'd talk I'd see her lips moving and not hear her speaking. I also remember watching my mother's mouth move and not hearing a word she was saying. She'd say to me, 'Repeat what I've just said,' but I couldn't."

"I wonder if she can do these things," Peter said to me, "because God endowed her with an unusually good brain or because of brain damage."

"Is there evidence of brain damage?" I asked.

"No, but her mother and grandmother said she'd been born prematurely and only weighed three or four pounds."

Her birth certificate showed she had been born at nine months, but if she had been born prematurely, she would have been more likely to have brain damage than a baby of normal weight, as follow-up studies of low-weight premature babies have established.

Another reason for considering brain damage was her recurrent experience of apparitions. A disorder of perception, such as a hallucination, may be the sole manifestation of a form of epilepsy called temporal-lobe epilepsy, and epilepsy can be an expression of brain damage. However, Ruth could control her apparitional experiences remarkably well, retain her normal awareness during them, and recall them in detail afterward, all of which are uncharacteristic of epileptics. Besides, there was no family history of epilepsy. It seemed probable we would find no brain damage, but Peter and I wanted to rule it out definitely.

The EEG is often abnormal in epilepsy, but Ruth's EEG was normal, even when a light was repetitively flashed at her eyes, which sometimes elicits an EEG abnormality that is not otherwise evident.

Ruth's performance was superior on two screening tests for brain damage in which she was presented with certain information and asked to recall it forty minutes or an hour later.[39] After the delay, people with brain damage, particularly temporal-lobe damage, usually display deficient recall. Vicky Rippere, who administered the tests, concluded that there was no evidence of impaired mental function. "Her brain is as clean as a whistle," Vicky said.

Ruth's computerized tomography scan was also normal. This is a new technique that X-rays the brain in multiple planes, outlines various brain structures very accurately, and can display minor degrees of brain damage. When Peter had found out the test result, Ruth asked him if it showed that her brain was normal.

"Normal," Peter said.

"Completely normal?" she asked.

"Not only is your brain normal, but it got up off the X-ray table to shake my hand so that I could congratulate it."

After these explorations, Peter and I concluded that Ruth had been endowed with an unusual brain and not a damaged one.

How had she managed to block her visual and auditory evoked responses? I told the results to Malcolm Lader, honorary consultant psychiatrist at the Maudsley Hospital. "She probably can do it," he said, "because of an unusually good capacity to focus her attention where she wants and exclude thereby things around her." This was consistent with Ruth's description of how she had done it.

Peter and I had her try several more times to block her evoked responses. We found that she varied considerably in her ability from one attempt to another and that her success sometimes seemed to depend on how much we encouraged her.

Apart from blocking Ruth's visual and auditory evoked responses, were there other measurable ways in which the apparitions affected her as a real person would?

Peter wet Ruth's forearm with methylated spirits, which evaporate quickly. He kneeled down next to her chair and blew on her forearm to speed the evaporation. The evaporation cooled her forearm, making its hair stand up.

"When I get home," Ruth said, "I'm going to enjoy telling my children how an English doctor got down on his knees and blew on my arm."

Peter laughed.

When the forearm warmed up again, the hairs lay flat.

Peter asked Ruth if an apparition could put methylated spirits on her forearm and blow on it.

A few seconds passed. "My arm feels cool now, Peter," she said. "I had my husband's apparition put that stuff on my arm and cool my arm by fanning it with a book."

I got on my knees, as Peter did, to look at the hairs. They were standing up—though not as much as when Peter had blown on her arm.

Ruth had produced a visible event that corresponded with her experience of her forearm becoming cool.

A few minutes later, I slapped Ruth's forearm hard enough to leave on it four red marks, where four fingers had hit her. Peter told the hospital photographer, whom he had invited to the experiment, to take pictures of the forearm fifteen, thirty, and forty-five seconds after the slap.

Peter asked Ruth to have an apparition slap her other arm and to signal the moment of the slap. She used an apparition of me. "That slap was too hard," she said to me in mock pain after the slap. "I'm going to hallucinate an apparition of Peter hitting you, so that you'll know what it feels like." Photographs were taken fiftten, thirty, and forty-five seconds after my apparition had slapped her.

Ruth had the apparition slap her a second time. After she signaled to us, Peter told her to intensify the feeling of pain in her arm. Again three pictures were taken of her arm.

All three pictures taken after I slapped Ruth showed her forearm to be reddened, whereas none of the six pictures taken after the two apparitional slaps did.

Before the experiment, I had wondered if an apparition's slap might leave bruises on her arm. If it did, perhaps the bruises she remembered having been left with at ten after her father's assault had resulted from an apparitional assault, though I did not regard this possibility seriously. In fact, the experiment left no bruises.

If she hallucinated the taste of a lemon on her tongue, would she salivate as if a real lemon were there?

Six times we put on her tongue three granules of citric acid, which gives lemons their taste; six times we asked her to hallucinate the taste of lemon; six times we asked her to imagine it; and six times we did not ask her to do anything. We tried each of the four conditions according to a random order, so that she did not know in advance which of the four conditions was coming up next. Twenty-four times we measured the amount she salivated, by comparing the weight of a fresh cotton swab before putting it under her tongue with its weight after being under her tongue for twenty seconds.

"How do you hallucinate the taste of lemon?" I asked her.

"I have Paul's apparition put citric acid granules that are on the end of its finger on my tongue, while I'm putting the swab under my tongue."

"And when you imagine the taste?" I asked.

"I just imagine it," she replied.

She salivated the most with the real citric acid granules, less when she hallucinated them, still less when she imagined them, and least when nothing was done. The difference between the amounts she salivated when imagining and when hallucinating the granules was more than two times greater than the difference between the amounts when tasting the real granules and when hallucinating them.

To compare her results with those of someone who lacked her talent, we repeated the experiment with me as the subject. Six times Peter put citric acid granules on my tongue, six times I imagined a lemon taste, and six times we did neither. The results showed that I salivated much more with the real lemon taste than with the imaginary one, and much more with the imaginary one than with nothing.

I salivated less with the real lemon taste than Ruth had in hallucinating it, even though in the "imagine" condition I salivated more than she had.

In summary, when hallucinating the citric acid granules, Ruth had salivated much more than when imagining them, less than when actually tasting them, and more than when I had actually tasted them.[40]

Could Ruth's eyes track the hallucinatory movement of a pendulum, as if it were actually moving?

Placed around Ruth's eyes were electrodes that were connected to pen and paper, so that her eye movements could be traced out.

As she watched a pendulum moving, her eyes displayed normal smooth tracking movements.

When asked to hallucinate the pendulum moving, she had an apparition of her daughter Heather pushing it. We then asked Ruth to imagine the pendulum moving.

In both the "hallucinate" and "imagine" conditions, Ruth's eyes failed to track the pendulum smoothly. As people who are sitting close to a tennis match where the ball is moving too fast for their eyes to follow it flick their eyes back and forth between the locations where they anticipate the ball will land, so she did between the locations where she judged a moving pendulum would reach the ends of its arc. In the "hallucinate" condition, her eyes flicked between locations that were more symmetrical with respect to the midline and remained more constant than in the "imagine" condition.

The result indicated that her eyes could smoothly track a real moving object, but not a hallucinatory or imaginary one. It meant, as Peter said, that the brain centers involved in producing smooth tracking movements could not be "conned."

At the Royal Marsden Hospital in London, Ruth tried to warm her right hand by having an apparition of her daughter place a hallucinatory heater in front of it. Ruth sat near a thermograph, a machine that measures the heat given off by the skin and displays warm skin on a television screen as dark and cold skin as light. On the screen, Peter and I watched her hands.

The room temperature was 60 degrees F, and before Ruth started to make the apparition, the television screen had shown the skin temperature of her hands to be about 82 degrees F.

Peter and I saw on the screen that her right hand stayed the same shade. However, after about two minutes, the fingertips of both hands began to darken on the screen, and over the next two minutes, they darkened more, Four minutes after Ruth had stopped hallucinating the heater, the screen showed that all ten of her fingertips were over 5 degrees F warmer than they had been before she had started.

As her right hand had not actually warmed in response to the hallucinatory heater, it was odd that all her fingertips had showed a delayed warming, as happens ordinarily after one hand has actually been warmed.

When her fingertips had cooled again to about 82 degrees F, we warmed her right hand with an actual heater. Her right hand quickly got darker on the screen, and lighter when we took the heater away. About two minutes later the fingertips of both hands began to darken. After four minutes they were as dark as they had been four minutes after she had tried to warm her right hand with a hallucinatory heater.

Could blood filling her fingertips have warmed them, because she had been holding her hands downward in front of the hallucinatory heater? We asked her to hold her fingers in that position for five minutes, but their temperature did not change. Why had all her fingertips showed the same delayed warming after she had hallucinated a heater in front of her right hand as after an actual heater had been there? This was an interesting question that would have to be explored later, since Ruth's stay in England was now ending.

"Well, I hope you learned something from all that," Ruth said to me as I drove her to Heathrow airport.

"I learned that your body and brain are likelier to respond to conjured-up phenomena as if they were real than most people's are," I said. "I also learned that your ability to do that has limits."

"Do you understand me any better now?"

I wondered if she was accusing me of being more interested in her abilities than in her.

"Yes," I said. "And I understand your abilities better. You're a very unusual person."

"Paul teases me about being a freak."

"Maybe he's envious."

"Are you?"

I shrugged my shoulders. "I think I've just accepted that you can do things that I can't."

"Where do we go from here?"

"How do you mean?"

"Are we going to do more experiments?"

"Do you want to?"

"Yes."

"I'm going to write up what's happened so far. After you and my colleagues have read it and responded to it, we'll see."

"It would make good material for a biography of me. I'd like to try writing one. I've wanted to be a writer for a long time."

That was news to me.

"I wish I could help you write it up," she said.

"Maybe you will write it up, and I'll just be an apparition writing under your command."

She laughed. "A lot of what's happened to me wouldn't have happened without you," she said. "So anything you write up won't be only about me. It'll also be about you. About the part you played in helping me and in teaching me about myself. It'll be about your discoveries."

She took a deep breath.

"This has all been quite an adventure for me," she said.

"And for me."

Viewpoints

RUTH was back in the United States, and I was left with my memories and notes, and a wish to understand her better. The more information I had gathered about her, the more mysteries had emerged.

One question that had been preoccupying me for a long time was why the crisis that had brought her to me had happened when it had. I considered that in the summer of 1976 her older daughter had been three years old, the age at which Ruth had first entered the children's home. Could being with her three-year-old daughter have reminded Ruth of when she was parted at three from her grandmother, and led her to relive the fearfulness and depression she had felt then? In 1976, Ruth's eldest child, George, had been seven. Could this have provoked Ruth's memory of herself at seven, when her father had returned to the family? Could that be why her father's apparition had entered her life when it had? I knew that emotional distress coinciding with one's offspring reaching ages at which certain major events occurred in one's own life are well known in psychiatric lore, but I could only guess about their possible relation to Ruth's recent crisis.

A colleague of mine, to whom I told Ruth's story, suggested that maybe Ruth had had an unconscious wish to leave Paul and their children, as her mother had left her and her brother and sister; that the father's apparition embodied Ruth's unconscious guilt, punishing her for the wish; and that her anxiety was expressing her fear of the wish. It was an imaginative interpretation, but there was no strong evidence that she had had such a wish.

Being honest with myself, I had to admit that despite all my work with her, I did not know why her crisis had begun when it had.

I found it interesting that without knowing the immediate causes of her crisis, I had been able to help her to emerge from it. How had her improvement come about? Because of her suffering, she had very much wanted her crisis to end, and had left her family and traveled several hours to come to the Arbours Crisis Centre. It is believed that no permanent resident of Lourdes has ever received one of the "miracle cures" reported to occur there, implying that the pilgrimage to Lourdes is somehow a necessary ingredient of the cure. Ruth's pilgrimage to London had expressed her determination to be helped and perhaps had represented for her a ritualistic step toward a cure.

When she had been at the Crisis Centre, my calling what we did "therapy"—I could have called it "an experiment in imagination"—had probably led her to expect improvement in her condition. My being a doctor and a psychotherapist may have strengthened her expectation. The success of her psychotherapy could have been partly due to her expecting success, but not entirely, since other people have had high expectations of psychotherapy and been disappointed.

My being a doctor could have contributed to the successful result of the therapy in another way. "I want to be a doctor's little girl," Ruth had told Anne Kilcoyne during a return in a memory trance to ten. Whether she had actually wanted this at ten I do not know, but apparently some child inside the adult Ruth still did. Her relationship with me represented a fulfillment, in a sense, of her wish.

I knew that therapy is sometimes talked about as if it were a well-charted procedure based upon scientifically established facts—and to a small extent it is. However, I also knew that like any human relationship, it is subject to unpredictability. In reviewing my experience of psychotherapy, I recognized that my understanding of why psychotherapy is sometimes effective and other times not was very incomplete.

Nevertheless my speculation went on about why I had succeeded with Ruth. I supposed that in allying with her against the apparition's interference in her life, I had helped her to deal with the aftereffects of her father's invasions into her life. In her childhood his invasions had been arbitrary and at his whim; in her psychotherapy we had bent his apparition to her will.

Had she created the apparition with a therapeutic purpose in mind, albeit an unconscious one? Could the apparition have manifested to impel her to seek help? It was an appealing idea.

What other meanings might the apparition be given? I remembered Ruth telling me of looking at Yvonne, aged fifteen months, and seeing her father's face upon Yvonne's, of hearing his laughter muffling Yvonne's crying, and of hesitating to reach out to Yvonne for fear of touching him. I felt that Ruth's experience could be expressing an intuition that her father had wanted to be her baby. It could also be representing an unconscious wish of Ruth to stifle Yvonne whom she was finding very demanding. Perhaps it was manifesting a feeling that her father had suppressed her own emotions as a child and imposed his desires upon her. It could also be reflecting Ruth's memory of her father's assault and his attempts to muffle her cries for help. Other experiences of her father's apparition were open to various interpretations based upon her memories of her father, her unconscious wishes, or her unconscious insights about herself or about him.

Why she had chosen an apparition as a vehicle for manifesting her memories, wishes, or insights I did not know. Had I been less interested in her apparitional experiences, she might have paid less attention to them herself. By dramatizing her emotional problems in the person of the apparition, she had allowed me an opportune means for gaining access to them.

I asked myself why she had remained averse to producing an apparition of her mother. "I don't want to make an apparition of her badly enough to try," Ruth had once said. "We can't get anything from her apparition that we can't get from anyone else's," she had said another time. I wondered if she had feelings toward her mother that she did not want to face, such as hatred or bitterness. If so, her psychotherapy, which had been so successful in dealing with her father's apparition, had possibly not gone far enough. I had said this to her, but she had remained disinclined to make an apparition of her mother. I felt I might have understood Ruth better if I had known more about her mother.

Given that she went on producing apparitions after the psychotherapy ended, had she returned to normality or learned to accept an abnormality? So far as "normal" means regular and usual, she had remained abnormal, though feeling much better about herself and recognizing that a talent is often uncommon and therefore abnormal. She had told me that when driving on her own, she sometimes put an apparition in the seat next to her for company, and that when bored at a party she sometimes conversed silently with an apparition.

Were the various unusual experiences that Ruth had undergone after meeting me expressions of one talent or of several? Because it seemed unlikely that a person could be gifted with several uncommon abilities, I supposed she had a single basic one. What was it?

Perhaps it was a capacity for suppressing or discounting her knowledge of what was real so as to experience something else. In Peter Fenwick's laboratory, while trying to block a flashing light with an apparition's head, Ruth had known that the light was really there. She had known she was looking at the light and had, nonetheless, managed to see her daughter's head. To feel a draft of cold air when an apparition had opened the bathroom door, Ruth had had to disregard her awareness that the door had remained closed. To feel an apparition lift her leg, she had had to refuse to notice the actual position of her leg. To experience herself as her father or as a little girl, she had had to ignore her knowledge of who and where she really was. Perhaps she had her unusual experiences because of being able to withdraw her attention from the recognition of certain obvious realities.

During some of her unusual experiences, she had only partially repudiated her knowledge of what was real. When she had first changed her reflected face in the mirror into her father's face, she had continued to feel her own feelings while feeling his. Only later had she been able "to let go more," she said, and "go completely into his feelings." When she had first entered a memory trance, she had remained aware of being an adult talking to me, while seeing herself as a little girl and feeling that girl's feelings. Only later had she lost consciousness of her adult self.

Before she had met me, her disavowal of what she knew to be real had been involuntary, as when she had looked at Paul and seen her father. Even while seeing her father, she had known it was Paul, but the knowledge had not prevented her from seeing her father. As the result of meeting me, she had learned to control this kind of phenomenon. She had come to see it as evidence of a skill, not of craziness.

Were there people who had had experiences similar to hers and had avoided psychiatrists for fear of being considered crazy? I recalled something a teacher of mine had once said: "Nature never creates just one instance of anything." So where were the other instances of this sort of phenomenon?[41]

I knew that when hypnotized some people can see someone who is not there, if the hypnotist suggests it.[42] But no one had ever hypnotized Ruth; she had never seen anyone hypnotized, as far as she knew; and she had never knowingly hypnotized herself. A few people can see things that are not there if someone tells them to, and a very few can do so at will, simply by deciding to.[43] It seemed that Ruth was one of these, since she could not recall anyone, except for me, having suggested to her that she see an apparition. How had she learned to do it?

As a child, her talking to dolls as if they were real and her having imaginary friends meant that she had felt comfortable in embellishing reality. A childhood capacity to produce eidetic images may have enabled her to make vivid the imaginary presence of people she knew.

I recalled Anne Kilcoyne having repeated something that Ruth had told her. "When my father got in a rage with me, Grandma used to tell me not to let his words touch me and to concentrate on a stream of beautiful feelings. After getting a beating from him, I'd lie down in the grass and concentrate on feeling the grass on my skin, and I'd stop feeling pain." Maybe Ruth had first learned and practiced some of her skills as strategems for dealing with unpleasant realities, and had been encouraged in doing so by her grandmother. Maybe in this way she had survived and surmounted difficulties that would have overpowered other children.

It occurred to me that her consent to the publication of her story may have also been a method of coping with unpleasant childhood realities. Adults in her family had repeatedly told her as a child not to disclose things about the family to any outsider, and she had complied. Now, though remaining anonymous, she was disclosing her history to anyone who cared to read it. A colleague of mine suggested that she may have been getting revenge on her family for the suffering they had caused her.

In my view the book probably meant many things to Ruth, and one of them was that it was a vehicle for announcing that she had overcome her shame and guilt about her past and herself.

On the inkblot test in her adult state, she had seen a butterfly coming out of a cocoon on one card. She was that butterfly, I thought. She had said that she was feeling hopeful about herself, more so than she ever had.

Was her hopefulness justified? A year after I had last seen her, which was two and a half years after our first meeting, I phoned her while I was in New York.

"Hi," I began, "I'm ringing to say the book is nearly finished."

"I'm looking forward to seeing it in bookstores."

"How've you been lately?"

"Well, nothing dramatic has been happening in my life. I'm happy with Paul and my children and myself. I'm less bothered than I used to be if someone says I weigh too much or recognizes me from the children's home."

She laughed.

"I'm laughing at myself for giving such silly examples of my happiness. It's hard to describe being happy, but I know I am." She lowered her voice. "One thing that makes me happy is that sex with Paul has been very good, better than it ever used to be."

"I'm very pleased. Have you been seeing any apparitions?"

"Yes. They're just entertainment for me now. I play with them. I haven't seen my father's apparition, thank goodness."

"How is your father?"

"He's in a bad way now, everyone says. It's his liver. He's in the hospital. They wanted to know if I'd go and spend time with him, but I said, 'Oh, no!'"

"And your mother?"

"As before. We aren't very close. Mainly I pity her. I've sometimes wondered why she played so small a part in our work together."

"Yes?"

"I compared myself to her, and realized I could never leave my children. I felt disappointed in her, and angry. Those feelings hadn't come out in me as a child, but they gradually seeped through the seams of my mind, and I felt guilty. If I'd made an apparition of her, I might have said, 'Hey, I hate you!' I didn't want to let that out. Yet somehow I did go through a period of hating her to get to where I am now."

"Where's that?"

"I had to climb a hill, and a lot of things were in my way. But I think I've reached the top."

"Have you got any ideas what brought on the crisis that you came to me with?"

"All the stuff inside me was buried so long, and just erupted or exploded. If something did trigger it, maybe it was my being overseas, without friends nearby, or maybe, as you've said, it was my children reaching certain ages and reminding me of myself at those ages. I'm pretty sure I'll never go through anything like I did in 1976."

"What makes you sure?"

"So many miseries of my growing-up years are out of my system, and once that's happened—well, it's happened. I don't have that burden anymore."

Neither of us said anything for a moment.

"I'd like to see the day," she said, "when people aren't as afraid as I was to share their strange experiences, even their unhappy ones. I hope the book will help bring that day about."

"So do I."

Notes

These notes consist of some thoughts I had while writing the book, references for the reader who wishes to explore further issues raised by the story, and numerical data, statistical analyses, and graphs to supplement my account of the experiments.

1. Between about 1893 and 1896 Freud held that hysteria resulted from sexual experiences in childhood: an assault by an adult stranger, a seduction by an adult close to the child, or sexual relations between two children. See Freud, "The Aetiology of Hysteria" (1896), in *The Standard Edition of the Complete Psychological Works of Sigmund Freud* (London: Hogarth, 1962), vol. III, pp. 191-221. Before Freud wrote this article, he had treated eighteen people with hysteria by psychoanalysis; all had told him they had had these kinds of childhood sexual experiences (ibid., pp. 207-8), and in two cases he had obtained confirmation of their assertions from other persons. Yet less than a year and a half later, he had retracted his conclusions; see the editor's footnote to Freud's "My Views on the Part Played by Sexuality in the Aetiology of the Neurosis" (1905), *Standard Edition,* vol. VII, p. 275.

2. For information about Arbours, write to 55 Dartmouth Park Road, London. NW5.

3. The study referred to is D. L. Rosenhan's "On Being Sane in Insane Places," *Science* 179 (January 19, 1973): 250-58.

4. The incidence of visual, auditory, and tactile hallucinatory experiences in mentally healthy people in England and Wales was surveyed between 1889 and 1892 by Henry Sidgwick et al.,

"Report of the Census of Hallucinations," *Proceedings of the Society for Psychical Research* 10 (1894): 25-422.

5. In mid-Wales, 137 widows and widowers out of 295 interviewed were found to have felt the presence of, seen, heard, spoken to, or been touched by the dead spouse. W. Dewi Rees, "The Hallucinations of Widowhood," *British Medical Journal* 4 (October 2, 1971): 37-41.

6. The Senoi approach to dreams is described by Kilton Stewart, "Dream Theory in Malaya," in Charles T. Tart (ed.), *Altered States of Consciousness: A Book of Readings* (New York and London: Wiley, 1969). That dreams may have played less part in Senoi life than Stewart reported is suggested by Richard Benjamin, "Temiar Religion," Cambridge Ph.D. thesis, and by Richard Bloch, "Report on a Trip to Malaysia," *East-West Journal,* October 1977.

7. A recurrent nightmare that was treated according to a principle similar to the one I used with this apparition is reported by Isaac M. Marks, "Rehearsal Relief of a Nightmare," *British Journal of Psychiatry* 133 (1978): 461–65.

8. A review of the treatment of phobias by means of exposure to the feared situation or object can be found in Isaac M. Marks, *Living With Fear: Understanding and Coping with Anxiety* (New York: McGraw-Hill, 1978).

9. A note on the usual harmlessness of exposure treatment is found in Marks, *Living with Fear,* p. 203.

10. Doctors in the United States label many more people schizophrenic than doctors do in most other countries. I think it likely that, outside the United States, Ruth's father would have received a different label, though I cannot say which one without having interviewed him.

11. Ruth's father's experience of hearing his doctor conclude that he was dead strikingly resembles a woman's experience quoted by Raymond A. Moody, Jr., *Life After Life* (Atlanta: Mockingbird Books, 1975), p. 26.

12. Stories of a person's apparition manifesting at the time or very near the time of that person's death were collected by Edmund Gurney, Frederic W. H. Myers, and Frank Podmore,

Phantasms of the Living, vols. I and II (London: Trübner, 1886); and by Eleanor Sidgwick, "Phantasms of the Living," *Proceedings of the Society for Psychical Research* 33 (1922).

13. Many events related in this book are open to psychological interpretations that I have not presented to the reader. For instance, Ruth's hallucinatory experience of two hospital orderlies putting her on a trolley could be interpreted as expressing her unconscious wish to miscarry the baby, and her difficulty in coping with the baby's demands months after it was born could be seen as corroborating that interpretation.

In order to preserve the continuity of the narrative, I have resisted the temptation to give more interpretations than I do.

14. Since 1838, when J. E. D. Esquirol, a French psychiatrist, gave the term "hallucination" its modern definition, it has meant the apparent perception of an object when no such object is present. Esquirol, *Des Maladies Mentales* (Paris: Ballière, 1838).

Some authors have given the name "pseudo-hallucination" to the experience of having a hallucination that one recognizes to be a hallucination; see G. Sedman, "A Comparative Study of Pseudo-Hallucinations, Imagery, and True Hallucinations," *British Journal of Psychiatry*, vol. 112, pp. 9–17. By this definition, Ruth's apparitional experiences were pseudohallucinations. However, since other authors have used the term "pseudohallucination" differently—for instance, to refer to an experience of an image that lacks the reality of a perception—I have not applied the term to Ruth's experiences. See E. H. Hare, "A Short Note on Pseudo-Hallucinations," *British Journal of Psychiatry*, vol. 122, pp. 469–76.

15. The characteristics of apparitions are presented and discussed in George N. M. Tyrrell, *Apparitions* (New York: Collier Books, 1963); and in Celia Green and Charles McCreery, *Apparitions* (London: Hamish Hamilton, 1975).

16. The quotation from C. D. Broad comes from his *Lectures on Psychical Research* (London: Routledge and Kegan Paul, 1962), pp. 253–54. Broad's book gives a thorough and critical account of the phenomenon of trance mediumship.

17. Much of what is known about dual and multiple person-

alities is reviewed in Ernest R. Hilgard, *Divided Consciousness: Multiple Controls in Human Thought and Action* (New York and London: Wiley, 1977).

18. In psychoanalytic idiom, the "father" of these trances can be considered an introject. "Introjection" refers to a normal process whereby a child takes into itself a representation or an image of a parent, which becomes a part of the child's self. See Roy Schafer, *Aspects of Internalization* (New York: International Universities Press, 1968), especially chaps. 4 and 5.

19. R. E. L. Masters, in *Eros and Evil: The Sexual Psychopathology of Witchcraft* (New York: Matrix House, 1966), "explores the sexual relations of humans with demons (incubi and succubi) as reported in the writings of witch-era scholars and those concerned with the apprehension and punishment of witches."

20. William H. Masters and Virginia E. Johnson, *Human Sexual Response* (Boston: Little, Brown, 1966). They did not find a woman capable of fantasying to orgasm, but they cite other investigators who had described such women, p. 134.

21. According to Sidgwick et al., "Report of the Census of Hallucinations," when more than one person was present while an apparition was being seen or heard, in about one-third of the cases it was seen or heard by more than one person. The figures documenting this statement are given by Tyrrell, *Apparitions,* pp. 24–5.

22. The phenomenon of imaginary companions in childhood is reviewed in Josephine R. Hilgard, *Personality and Hypnosis: A Study of Imaginative Involvement* (Chicago: University of Chicago Press, 1970), chap. 10.

23. The possibility that an adult can recollect birth or prebirth experiences is viewed favorably by R. D. Laing in *The Facts of Life* (New York: Pantheon, 1976), chap. 5.

24. Months after the inkblot testing I told Anne Kilcoyne that I planned to publish the test results in a book. When I said that I had in mind to reproduce in the book some of the inkblots, she objected. She pointed out that if members of the public had access to the inkblots, they could rehearse their responses to them before being tested.

I discussed the matter with other colleagues. One psychologist, who often administered the inkblot test, opposed my publishing them for the same reason Anne did. Other psychologists felt differently. "Anyone can find out what typical responses to the inkblots are by looking in psychology texts," said one psychologist. "I'd publish the inkblots if I were you." Another psychologist said, "So many influences already affect test subjects' responses, such as the circumstances in which the test is given, the subject's opinion about the purposes of the testing, and the psychologist's behavior during the testing. Subjects seeing the inkblots in advance will make little difference."

I considered the arguments carefully. I felt sympathy with Anne's objection, but thought the public's right to knowledge superseded some psychologists' interests in keeping that knowledge privileged. As I wanted to illustrate Ruth's responses to the inkblots, I decided to publish them. The facsimiles reproduced here came from my own set of inkblots, and the indications of where on the inkblots Ruth had seen the things she did came from notes I had made during the testing.

25. The phenomenon of hypnotic age regression is probed in Robert Reiff and Martin Scheerer, *Memory and Hypnotic Age Regression: Developmental Aspects of Cognitive Function Explored Through Hypnosis* (New York: International Universities Press, 1959); and in Ernest R. Hilgard's *Divided Consciousness,* chap. 3.

26. The Semantic Differential is described in detail in C. E. Osgood, G. J. Suci, and P. H. Tannenbaum, *The Measurement of Meaning* (Urbana: University of Illinois Press, 1957). Osgood and Zella Luria applied it to the personalities of Eve, "A Blind Analysis of a Case of Multiple Personality Using the Semantic Differential," *The Journal of Abnormal and Social Psychology* 49 (1954): 579–91. Osgood, Luria, R. F. Jeans, and S. W. Smith applied it to another case of multiple personality, "The Three Faces of Evelyn: A Case Report," *Journal of Abnormal Psychology* 85 (1976): 247–86.

27. References for the Twenty Statements Test are Manford H. Kuhn and Thomas S. McPartland, "An Empirical Investigation of Self-Attitudes," *The American Sociological Review* 19

(1954): 68–76; and Kuhn, "Self-Attitudes by Age, Sex, and Professional Training," *Sociological Quarterly* 1 (1960): 39–55.

28. In giving the results of the Semantic Differential, I indicate by the number 7 if Ruth marked the space nearest to "valuable," 6 if she marked the space next to that space, 5 if she marked the next space, 4 if she marked the middle space between "valuable" and "worthless," and so on, until 1 if she marked the space nearest to "worthless." Similarly, I indicate by 7 if she marked the space next to "deep," "fast," "active," "large," "clean," "strong," "tasty," "relaxed," or "hot"; and by 1 if she marked the space next to "shallow," "slow," "passive," "small," "dirty," "weak," "distasteful," "tense," or "cold." [See chart on facing page.]

29. The responses given by Ruth's normal adult self and by the apparition of herself differed on five of the ten scales, and three of these differences were greater than one scale point (5, 3, 3). Analysis of the data for significance of differences using the Wilcoxon matched-pairs signed-ranks test yielded a nonsignificant result ($T = 5$, $N = 5$, N.S.). The Sign test and the McNemar test for the significance of changes gave similar results. These statistical tests are described in Sidney Siegel, *Nonparametric Statistics for the Behavioural Sciences* (New York and London: McGraw-Hill, 1956).

30. The results at fifteen in the "imagine" condition and in the memory trance differed in seven of the ten scales. In the trance at ten, she wrote responses on only four of the ten scales, and three of these four differed from the corresponding responses in the "imagine" condition.

Vicky Rippere thought it was justified to combine these two sets of data, because we had no reason to suppose that either trance personality was less genuine than the other, especially since each personality's responses differed in about the same percentage of cases (70 percent and 75 percent) from those in the corresponding "imagine" condition. Of the 11 differences between the two sets of "imagine" and trance responses, 10 were greater than one scale point, the average difference being 4.22. Analysis of the results for significance of differences using the Wilcoxon test was highly

	Normal Adult Self	Apparition of Self	"Imagine" at 15	Memory Trance at 15	"Imagine" at 10	Memory Trance at 10
Valuable-worthless	7	7	6	7	5	—
Deep-shallow	7	7	5	7	4	—
Fast-slow	2	7	1	7	7	7
Active-passive	7	6	7	7	4	7
Large-small	6	7	1	7	1	7
Clean-dirty	7	7	4	4	4	—
Strong-weak	4	7	2	7	4	7
Tasty-distasteful	7	7	2	7	5	—
Relaxed-tense	4	4	2	4	4	—
Hot-cold	7	4	1	1	4	—

significant this time. ($T = 0$, $N = 10$, p.$<.01$ two-tailed; a two-tailed test was used, because a direction of difference had not been predicted.)

If the two sets of data are left uncombined, and the responses in the trance at fifteen are compared with those in the "imagine" condition at fifteen, the differences are statistically significant ($T = 0$, $N = 7$, p$<.02$ two-tailed).

In the Twenty Statements Test, when imagining herself at fifteen, Ruth wrote:

1. I am shy.
2. I am afraid.
3. I am witty.
4. I am in love.
5. I am hate.
6. I am alone.
7. I am a girl.
8. I am determined.
9. I am important to someone.
10. I am a swimmer.
11. I am an excellent skater.
12. I am what I am.

When imagining herself at ten, she wrote:

1. I am my name.
2. I am a sister.
3. I am a granddaughter.
4. I am a daughter.
5. I am a niece.
6. I am Becky's friend.
7. I am a schoolgirl.
8. I am a baby-sitter.
9. I am an almost teenager.
10. I am thin.
11. I am a fast runner.
12. I am a good bike rider.

31. The phenomenon of eidetic imagery is described by Ralph Norman Haber, "Eidetic Images," *Scientific American* 220 (April 1969): 36–44, and the picture of the Rogues' Gallery is taken from that article. The phenomenon is also reviewed in Ian M. L. Hunter, *Memory* (Harmondsworth and New York: Penguin Books), pp. 195–204; and its frequency is discussed in R. N. Haber and R. B. Haber, "Eidetic Imagery: 1. Frequency," *Perceptual and Motor Skills* 19 (1964): 131–38.

32. Old Blind Mole was drawn by Alan Aldridge and appears as plate 3 in Aldridge and William Plummer, *The Butterfly Ball* (London: Jonathan Cape, 1973).

33. The test administered by Nick Stirling was the Stroop color-word test. John Ridley Stroop, "Studies of Interference in Serial Verbal Reactions," *Journal of Experimental Psychology* 18 (1935): 643–62.

34. Here, in milliseconds, are the mean vocal reaction times and the standard deviations for the "agree" and "disagree" conditions in each of the three states:

| | "Agree" | | "Disagree" | |
	Mean	SD	Mean	SD
Memory trance, age three	1280	397	1139	187
Memory trance, age seven	1207	370	882	194
Normal adult, age twenty-seven	803	195	1162	380

In the normal adult state her responses were faster to a statistically significant degree in the "agree" than in the "disagree" condition (t_{31} = 3.162, p<.01).

In the memory trance at age three, the two sets of responses did not differ to a statistically significant degree (t_{32} = 1.295, p<0.1). In the memory trance at age seven, the two sets of responses did differ to a statistically significant degree (t_{31} = 12.784, p<.001), but in the reverse direction from the difference in the adult state.

35. That there is sometimes no interference effect during the transition stage from nonreader to reader is suggested by R. Friedman, "The Relationship Between Intelligence and Performance on the Stroop Color-Word Test in Second- and Fifth-

Grade Children," *The Journal of Genetic Psychology* 118 (1971): 147–48.

36. Possibly, Ruth's being in a trance state was itself associated with the blocking of the interference effect in the "disagree" condition, though there is no obvious reason why it should be. We could have tested this possibility by asking her to return in a memory trance to an age when she would have been expected to show an interference effect, such as fifteen.

37. The use of evoked responses in investigating hysterical symptoms is reviewed by Malcolm Lader, *The Psychophysiology of Mental Illness* (London: Routledge and Kegan Paul, 1975), pp. 190–92. Lader says (p. 192): "In view of the complex and unclear relationships between hysteria and hypnosis, it is appropriate to mention that no consistent, unequivocal effects of hypnotic suggestion have ever been demonstrated in an adequate number of subjects, although there have been interesting individual cases in which marked attenuation of the evoked response occurred when the suggestion was made under hypnosis that the stimulus was absent."

38. These are the tracings of our experiments with Ruth's visual and auditory evoked responses:

Flash evoked response — 16 trials

The visual evoked response to sixteen pattern reversals averaged and recorded from an electrode 5 cm above the inion referred to the vertex.

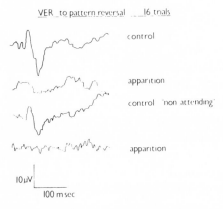

The mean visual evoked reponse to a flash stimulus averaged over sixteen trials recorded from an electrode 5 cm above the inion referred to the vertex.

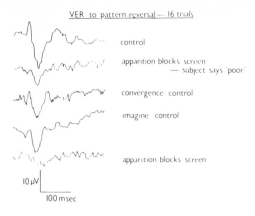

The visual evoked response to sixteen pattern reversals averaged and recorded from an electrode 5 cm above the inion referred to the vertex.

Auditory evoked response — 32 trials

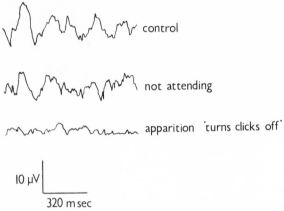

The mean of thirty-two trials to a medium-intensity click stimulus recorded from C2 to the right mastoid.

39. To screen Ruth for brain damage Vicky Rippere used two tests of short-term and long-term recall. On the Wechsler Logical Memory test Form I, Vicky read to Ruth two passages labeled A and B. She then asked Ruth to repeat to her as much of the passages as Ruth could. The number of bits Ruth could remember was her score, and that number divided by the total number of bits was her percent recall. An hour later, Vicky asked her again to repeat the passage. The results were:

Immediate recall   A = 13 B = 11   % recall = 52.17%
Delayed recall   A = 11 B = 11   % recall = 47.83%
      Delayed/Immediate recall = 91.66%

Ruth's score placed her clearly in the non-brain-damaged category.

On the Rey-Osterrieth Form II test, after letting Ruth see a complex drawing, Vicky took it away and asked Ruth to draw as much of it as she could from memory. Forty minutes later, she asked Ruth to draw it again. The maximum possible score is 45. Ruth's score was 45 on immediate recall and 34 after forty minutes, both of which are very superior.

40. In the lemon-tasting experiment, the mean weight gains of the swabs and the standard deviations were as follows:

RUTH

	Granules of Citric Acid (L_R)	Hallucinate (H_R)	Imagine (I_R)	Nothing (Control) (C_R)
Mean weight gain	1879	1495	565	374
Standard deviation	278	327	159	147

L_R vs. H_R $t = -2.18$ $p = 0.05$
H_R vs. I_R $t = 6.25$ $p = 0.0001$
I_R vs. C_R $t = -2.16$ $p = 0.06$
H_R vs. C_R $t = 7.65$ $p = 0.00002$

MORTY

	Granules of Citric Acid	Imagine	Nothing (Control)
Mean weight gain	1180	632	210
Standard deviation	256	114	190

41. A book by a nineteenth-century physician, W. B. Carpenter, describes the phenomenon of "Spectral Illusions," which are "mental images" that resemble "the creations of dreaming or delirium" except that they "mingle with the sensations called forth by objective realities."

Carpenter cites from Dr. Abercombie (*Inquiries Concerning the Intellectual Powers,* 5th ed., p. 382) the case of a "gentleman who was all his life haunted by Spectral figures, and could call up any at will, by directing his attention steadily to some conception of his own mind, which might either consist of a figure or a scene that he had seen, or might be a composition of his own imagination: but although possessing the faculty of producing the illusion, he had no power of banishing it. . . ."

Carpenter describes another case in which a man had "the

same Sensorial condition as in dreaming or delirium," which was "accompanied by an Intellectual recognition of its objective unreality." Carpenter says that the man "was perfectly healthy, his mind was of more than ordinary strength, and he would speak of his phantoms. and reason upon their appearance. . . ." Carpenter, *Principles of Mental Physiology*, 6th ed. (London: C. Kegan & Co., 1881), pp. 164–67.

42. Much about Ruth's case can be related to hypnotic phenomena. Fred H. Frankel and Martin T. Orne found that a group of phobic patients, especially those with multiple phobias, displayed a high degree of hypnotizability; "Hypnotizability and Phobic Behaviour," *Archives of General Psychiatry*, Vol. 33, October 1976, pp. 1259–1261. The authors suggest that these patients' hypnotizability rendered them vulnerable to developing phobias in the course of spontaneously occurring trance-like states. The authors recommend treating such individuals by hypnotizing them and inducing them to have experiences that closely resemble their symptoms. In this way the patient can experience "feelings previously seen as frightening and ego alien as familiar, under his control, and perhaps even as comfortable" (p. 1261).

43. Many physicians, including Jean-Martin Charcot, Pierre Janet, and Joseph Breuer, have linked hypnotic phenomena with hysterical symptoms; see David Spiegel and Robert Fink, "Hysterical Psychosis and Hypnotizability," *American Journal of Psychiatry*, Vol. 136, No. 6, June 1979, pp. 777–81. Spiegel and Fink propose that some hysterical symptoms, such as hallucinations, can be "understood as spontaneous undisciplined trance states" occurring in individuals who are very easily hypnotized. In a remark possibly applicable to Ruth, the authors note that some hysterical symptoms "may be attributable to identification with a psychotic person close to the subject. This proneness to identification is a recognizable part of the syndrome of high hypnotizability . . ." (p. 778). They report using the trance capacity of two patients to demonstrate to the patients "their ability to bring on their own symptoms and thereby to master them" (p.780).